Clinical Hypnosis and Memory: Guidelines For Clinicians and For Forensic Hypnosis

by
D. Corydon Hammond, Ph.D., Richard B. Garver, Ed.D.,
Charles B. Mutter, M.D., Harold B. Crasilneck, Ph.D.,
Edward Frischholz, Ph.D., Melvin A. Gravitz, Ph.D.,
Neil S. Hibler, Ph.D., Jean Olson, MSN, RN, CS,
Alan Scheflin, J.D., LLM, Herbert Spiegel, M.D.,
and William Wester, Ed.D.

First Printing, February 1995

American Society
of Clinical Hypnosis Press

This publication has been created by members of the Hypnosis and Memory Committee of the American Society of Clinical Hypnosis, who are solely responsible for its content. All opinions expressed herein are those of the authors. It should be remembered that the appropriate treatment in any given situation will be largely dependent upon the specific facts and circumstances involved in that situation. Accordingly, the American Society of Clinical Hypnosis and the American Society of Clinical Hypnosis Press disclaim any and all warranties, express or implied, regarding any use or misuse of the information contained in this publication.

Manufactured in the United States of America

Library of Congress Cataloging-in-Publication Data
Clinical hypnosis and memory : guidelines for clinicians and for forensic hypnosis / by D. Corydon Hammond... [et al.].
p. cm.
Includes bibliographical references (p.).
ISBN 1-886610-01-0
1. Hypnotism -- Therepeutic use -- Standards. 2. Forensic hypnotism-Standards. 3. Memory. 4. Repression (Psychology) 5. Repression (Psychology) I. Hammond, D. Corydon. II. American Society of Clinical Hypnosis.
RC495.C532 1995
616.89' 162--dc20

95-6572
CIP

TABLE OF CONTENTS

INTRODUCTION

The American Society of Clinical Hypnosis (ASCH) is the largest professional scientific society and certifying body of licensed health and mental health care practitioners using hypnosis in North America. One of the Society's purposes is to set high standards for training and practice in the field of clinical hypnosis. The ASCH is committed to scientifically assessing all potential applications of hypnosis. Considerable research has been published on the topic of hypnosis and memory since the AMA Scientific Report in 1985. Criticisms have also appeared about the validity of the AMA report conclusions (Beahrs, 1988; Reiser, 1986; Rock v. Arkansas, 1987; Scheflin & Shapiro, 1989; Spiegel, 1987; Spiegel & Spiegel, 1987; Watkins, 1989). The AMA report was also limited in its scope to examining laboratory research and suggesting guidelines for forensic work. Therefore, the Executive Committee of the ASCH established a committee, which included three members of the original AMA panel. The objectives of the committee included exploring and evaluating both the older and more current scientific and clinical data on the nature of memory, the role of hypnosis in accessing memory, and the current status of the law concerning hypnosis and memory. The committee critically evaluated and reviewed research findings concerning hypnosis and memory, and subsequently created two sets of recommendations, one for licensed therapists using clinical hypnosis and updated recommendations for the conduct of forensic hypnosis interviews.

The interdisciplinary committee involved in evaluating the literature and preparing this report consisted of Richard B. Garver, Ed.D., ABPH, Co-Chair; Charles B. Mutter, M.D., ABMH, Co-Chair; D. Corydon Hammond, Ph.D., ABPH, Coordinator; Harold B. Crasilneck, Ph.D., ABPH, Edward Frischholz, Ph.D., Melvin A. Gravitz, Ph.D., ABPH, Neil S. Hibler, Ph.D., Jean Olson, MSN, RN, CS, Alan Scheflin, J.D., LLM, Herbert Spiegel, M.D., and William Wester, Ed.D., ABPH. The authors have donated all royalties from the sale of this document to the American Society of Clinical Hypnosis, which financially supported this expensive project.

After many months of work, an earlier draft of our report was sent to many national and international specialists and authorities in the fields of memory research, hypnosis, trauma treatment and research, and the law. About two-thirds of them took the time to provide us with feedback. We are grateful for their generosity and responsiveness to our requests for consultation. Their reactions were usually quite favorable, and their critical feedback furthered our insight into complex issues. Our consultants were invaluable in assisting us to achieve a balanced perspective and in creating an evenhanded document that takes into account biases and limitations in scientific research paradigms and in individual viewpoints. The committee made a sincere effort to synthesize and examine empirical findings in an intellectually honest manner and to avoid excesses or the taking of extreme or limited positions that are sometimes associated with single, circumscribed theoretical orientations in the fields of memory and hypnosis.

We extend our gratitude to Ernest R. Hilgard, Ph.D., David Spiegel, M.D., John G. Watkins, Ph.D., Erika Fromm, Ph.D., Jean Holroyd, Ph.D., Kevin M. McConkey, Ph.D., Daniel Brown, Ph.D., Steven Jay Lynn, Ph.D., Peter Bloom, M.D., Andre Weitzenhoffer, Ph.D., Fred H. Frankel, M.D., Frederick J. Evans, Ph.D., Helen Pettinati, Ph.D., Elizabeth Loftus, Ph.D., Sven-Ake Christianson, Ph.D., John Yuille, Ph.D., Bessel A. van der Kolk, M.D., Jennifer J. Freyd, Ph.D., Richard P. Kluft, M.D., Ph.D., Joan Turkus, M.D., Christine A. Courtois, Ph.D., Thurman Mott, M.D., Richard Horevitz, Ph.D., Joan Murray-Jobsis, Ph.D., Dabney Ewin, M.D., Gary R. Elkins, Ph.D., Michael J. Diamond, Ph.D., Irving Kirsch, Ph.D., Valerie J. Wall, Ph.D., Clorinda Margolis, Ph.D., Moshe Torem, M.D., Michael A. Haberman, M.D., Marlene Steinberg, M.D., Sheldon B. Cohen, M.D., Louis L. Dubin, D.D.S., Ph.D., Alvin Scott, Ph.D., J. Michael Marcum, M.D., Ph.D., Donald W. Schafer, M.D., O. Brandt Caudill, Jr., Michael D. Yapko, Ph.D., and Jordan Zarren, MSW.

Definition of Hypnosis

The term hypnosis was first used in the 1820's and it was soon identified as "controlled imagination" (Gravitz, 1993). Since then, there have been a variety of different definitions of hypnosis based upon various theoretical and research orientations (Lynn & Rhue, 1991), many of which are reflected by members of our committee. Many of the existing "theories" of hypnosis are descriptive rather than explanatory concerning hypnosis. Much of the apparent divergence among various definitions has centered around three basic issues: 1) features of hypnosis; 2) state/trait concepts; and 3) contextual factors.

Regarding the diversity of opinions about the nature of hypnosis, a large number of the definitions refer to three concurrent, overlapping components. Wide individual differences are found in each of these components, and it has been suggested that all three should be present in some degree to identify hypnosis (Spiegel & Greenleaf, 1992). Although sometimes referred to with different labels, these three components are: 1) dissociation; 2) absorption; and 3) suggestibility. Thus, we see, for example, that dissociation is sometimes referred to as involuntariness, unconscious response, or levels of consciousness (e.g., Bowers & Davidson, 1991; Crasilneck & Hall, 1985; Erickson, 1980; Hilgard, 1978, 1986; Watkins & Watkins, 1979-1980, 1981; Weitzenhoffer, 1989). Others emphasizing this general concept discuss alterations in brain processes (e.g., Crasilneck, McCranie, & Jenkins, 1956; Crawford & Gruzelier, 1992; DeBenedittis & Sironi, 1986, 1988; DePascalis & Penna, 1990; Rossi, 1993). Likewise, absorption (Tellegen, 1979) has also been referred to as imaginative involvement (Hilgard, 1970), focused concentration (Spiegel & Spiegel, 1978), and imagery vividness (Spanos, Brett, Menary, & Cross, 1987). Suggestibility

(Hull, 1933; Weitzenhoffer, 1953) has often been alluded to as a "suspension of critical judgement" (Hilgard, 1965; Kline, 1958; Meares, 1961; Orne, 1977).

Another area of debate concerning the nature of hypnosis has to do with the disagreement over whether hypnosis is defined as involving an altered state of consciousness (e.g., Fromm, 1992; Hilgard, 1977/1986, 1992; Spiegel & Spiegel, 1978), or is defined in terms of social psychological variables (Spanos & Chaves, 1989) such as expectations (Kirsch, 1991), role taking (Coe & Sarbin, 1991), compliance (Wagstaff, 1991), and contextual factors. As a way of avoiding theoretical conflicts over whether hypnosis involves an altered state, some persons have preferred to define hypnosis according to what occurs in hypnosis (Spiegel, 1963). Thus, it has been defined as a procedure wherein alterations in sensations, perceptions, feelings or behavior may be suggested.

Certainly, situational factors, demand characteristics, expectancies, goal-directed role playing or believed-in imagining, and motivation are all contextual issues which influence the degree to which individuals tap their capacity for hypnosis. With so many interactive features determining behavioral and subjective responses, it is important to make distinctions between external influences, phenomenology, reports of the subject, technique, therapeutic strategy, theoretical and clinical orientation of the therapist, and differences in potential for a given individual to experience hypnosis.

The courts have leaned toward defining hypnosis in terms of its antecedents, i.e., whether or not a hypnotic induction ceremony was administered (Scheflin & Shapiro, 1989). Unfortunately, this has downplayed the importance of defining hypnosis by its consequences (i.e., hypnotizability). The committee agrees that there are wide individual differences in responsivity to hypnosis, and that hypnotic response may also occur spontaneously or through informal encouragement, without the presence of a formal induction. It seems logical, then, that the court's definition of hypnosis in terms of whether or not an induction ceremony has been administered is problematic (Scheflin, 1994b). We believe that it should be demonstrated that both a hypnotic induction was administered, and that the subject was responsive to such a procedure (e.g., through the elicitation of phenomena either informally, or formally through the administration of a hypnotizability scale).

SECTION 1

CURRENT CONCEPTS ABOUT MEMORY AND FACTORS INFLUENCING MEMORY

Understanding the limitations of current scientific knowledge and after reviewing the large body of current research on memory we believe that, in brief, the following conclusions are currently justified.

Literature on normal memory (e.g., partially summarized by Loftus, 1993; Munsterberg, 1908) demonstrates that memory may be imperfect, adaptive and reconstructive rather than reproductive, and documents the potential malleability (Spiegel, 1974) of normal memory. Some degree of memory alteration appears to inevitably occur as part of daily living (Bartlett, 1932). The request that a person provide information about the past is always to some extent suggestive, whether the request is made in therapy, for forensic purposes, or otherwise (Spiegel, 1980). Furthermore, individual differences exist in the capacity to remember for a variety of reasons. But a balanced and accurate understanding of memory processes also requires one to be aware that research likewise strongly demonstrates that emotional memories may be encoded differently and be relatively accurate and persistent with regard to central details, which seem better retained and less susceptible to forgetting (e.g., Christianson, 1992c, 1992d).

In addition, the scientific community itself is divided as to whether memory is a unitary phenomenon, or whether unique subsystems of memory exist that perform specific functions, and there are over twenty different theories of memory that have been proposed. Some of the literature describes this as state-dependent (Bower, 1981; Tulving & Thomson, 1973), sensory-motor or somatic (Piaget, 1954), explicit or implicit (Schacter, 1987), episodic or semantic memory (Tulving, 1972). There does seem to be relative agreement that there are three phases to the memory process: encoding, storage and retrieval (e.g., Loftus, 1979). Memory may be influenced by problems during any one of these three phases, and by a variety of memory principles (Kihlstrom, 1994).

The committee wishes to emphasize that research focused on malleability of normal memory teaches us that there is potential for inaccuracy of recall of details, whether or not enhancement procedures have been used, so that the total accuracy of a memory cannot be claimed or assumed unless the memory is corroborated by independent sources and methods. At the same time, however, other simulation and autobiographical memory research has shown that there is often considerable accuracy of memory, especially in the recall of emotional/traumatic events. Thus, it seems imperative for professionals to take a balanced view of memory and not become influenced by extreme positions that represent an overgeneralization from studies of normal, unstressed memory processes.

We believe that just such a balanced position was what was taken this year by the American Psychiatric Association (1994) in their statement on memories of sexual abuse. On the one hand, they affirmed the existence of repressed and delayed memories, saying: "Children and adolescents who have been abused cope with the trauma by using a variety of psychological mechanisms. In some instances, these coping mechanisms result in a lack of conscious awareness of the abuse for varying periods of time. Conscious thoughts and feelings stemming from the abuse may emerge at a later date" (p. 26). At the same time, they emphasized that memory is a complex process, influenced by questioning, and that may include some false or contradictory elements. However, they added that "hesitancy in making a report, and recanting following the report can occur in victims of documented abuse. Therefore, these seemingly contradictory findings do not exclude the possibility that the report is based on a true event" (p. 24). Similar to the recommendations that follow in Section 3, they emphasized maintaining an empathic stance toward patients alleging abuse, and avoidance of prejudging the veracity of memories or that the memories are or are not the cause of symptoms. They stressed that expressing disbelief in patient symptoms could cause harm, and the importance of cautioning the patient against making major life decisions when in the acute phase of treatment. They also emphasized that special knowledge and experience are needed in working with patients who report the emergence of memories through the use of hypnosis.

The American Medical Association Council on Scientific Affairs (1994) has likewise issued a report on memories of childhood abuse. They noted that professionals may be found on both sides of the false memory issue. It was observed that "repeated questioning may lead individuals to report events that in fact never occurred" (p. 3). But, in addition to noting that memory may be flawed, they also acknowledged the existence of repressed memories: "Notwithstanding these findings, other research indicates that some survivors of abuse do not remember, at least temporarily, having been abused.... In short, empirical evidence can be cited for both sides of the argument. While virtually all would agree that memories are malleable and not necessarily fully accurate, there is no consensus about the extent or sources of this malleability. The issue is far from settled, and under such circumstances, therapists should exercise care in treating their patients, maintaining an empathic and supportive posture" (p. 3). Their final conclusion was that "the AMA considers recovered memories of childhood sexual abuse to be of uncertain authenticity, which should be subject to external verification" (p. 4); a conclusion mirrored by this committee.

In their report, the AMA quoted and reaffirmed their 1984 recommendations concerning the use of hypnosis in forensic (not clinical) settings with witnesses and victims of crimes, emphasizing the importance of guidelines similar to those elaborated in the last section of this volume. The report, however, reaffirmed as an accurate summary of the empirical literature, the limited perspective of their decade old policy that "hypnosis-induced recollections actually appear to be less reliable than nonhypnotic recall" (p. 2). As will be noted in the remainder of this volume, we disagree with this item in the AMA report. While their 1984 statement and 1985 report may have accurately reported laboratory research on normal memory (often for nonmeaningful material), it would be a violation of basic research standards to generalize and draw conclusions from one population to an entirely different population. Just as one cannot overgeneralize that a poll of college freshmen is predictive of how the general electorate will vote in a national election, so it is inappropriate to overgeneralize from laboratory studies of normal memory to a clinical population of abuse victims with emotion-laden, traumatic memories.

Traumatic Memory

The evidence from numerous real life and simulation studies suggests that traumatic memory appears different from the relatively unstressed memory processes often studied in laboratories. Traumatic memories may be encoded differently due to both attentional and psychological variables, as well as physiological factors (Cahill, Prins, Weber, & McGaugh, 1994; Christianson, 1992a; Horowitz & Reidbord, 1992; LeDoux, 1992, 1994); McGaugh, 1992; Nilsson & Archer, 1992; Pitman, 1994; Saporta & van der Kolk, 1992; van der Kolk, 1984, 1987, 1988; van der Kolk & Saporta, 1993; van der Kolk & Van der Hart, 1991; Weinberger, Gold, & Sternberg, 1984).

Thus, for example, van der Kolk (van der Kolk & van der Hart, 1991) notes that while memory is usually active and constructive, in cases involving PTSD, a failure of declarative memory may lead to organization of the trauma on a somatosensory level in the form of visual images or physical sensations that may be relatively impervious to change, a concept supported by Terr (1988). The committee recognizes that a major finding in both recent experimental studies and the clinical literature is that traumatic or emotion-laden memories tend to be accurate and persistent concerning the traumatic, critical details (Christianson, 1992b), although accessibility and accuracy of traumatic memories may be potentially influenced by other conscious, unconscious or physiologic factors (e.g., state-dependent context, motivation, secondary gain, phase of posttraumatic stress disorder, and interrogation methods).

There is also evidence that emotional memories are fairly consistent (though not necessarily always fully accurate) over time (Bohannon, 1990; Pillemer, 1984; Yuille & Cutshall, 1986), and that the degree of affect is predictive of the stability of memory (Bohannon, 1990; Pillemer, 1984). Victims of actual crimes (e.g., bank robberies) have been found to have greater accuracy of memory than bystander witnesses (e.g., customers) concerning central critical details, but less accuracy for peripheral, more irrelevant details (Christianson & Hubinette, 1993; Read, Yuille, & Tollestrup, 1992), a finding consistent with other laboratory research (summarized in Christianson, 1992b). These findings support the concept that memory for negative emotional events may be encoded differently than ordinary memory, perhaps through different attentional focusing, perhaps because of the distinctiveness of some emotional events, and perhaps because emotional arousal slows forgetting (Heuer & Reisberg, 1992), or some combination of these variables along with physiological factors. Research with children (e.g., Goodman, Hirschman, Heeps, & Rudy, 1991; Jones & Krugman, 1986; Ornstein, Gordon, Baker-Ward, & Merrit, in press; Terr, 1990; Warren & Swartwood, 1992) likewise documents the same pattern that is found in adult laboratory and real-life studies: children tend to remember critical details of traumatic events very well. And although children's memories of real events may certainly be influenced by misleading suggestions (e.g., Bruck, Ceci, Francouer, & Barr, in press; Ornstein, Gordon, & Baker-Ward, in press), seldom does a single suggestion concerning an important, personal autobiographical event influence the child's report (e.g., Rudy & Goodman, 1991; Saywitz, Goodman, Nicholas, & Moan, 1991).

However, an incomplete processing of emotional and cognitive material may be associated with a dose-related effect of trauma (Briere & Conte, 1993; Feldman-Summers & Pope, 1994; Herman & Schatzow, 1987; Shore, Tatum, & Vollmer, 1986, van der Kolk, Vardi, Eisler, Nerron, Hostettler, & Zakai, 1994)--that is, more intense, violent, or life threatening (or perceived as life threatening) trauma, or more than one type of abuse (e.g., physical and sexual) appears positively correlated with dissociation or amnesia for the traumatic event. Feldman-Summers and Pope (1994) discovered that 83% of psychologists who had been abused both physically and sexually reported periods of forgetting their abuse, while only 35% and 23%, respectively, of those who were only sexually abused or physically abused reported a period where they forgot some or all of their abuse. Interestingly, even soon after crimes, police have found that injured victims of crimes provide less information to investigators than noninjured victims, and victims of rape or assault provide less detailed descriptions than victims of robberies (Kuehn, 1974).

Relatedly, there exists abundant evidence for amnesia of traumatic events in a wide range of life circumstances (e.g. Coons, 1992; Coons & Milstein, 1990; Hilgard, 1986; Loewenstein, 1991; Schacter & Kihlstrom, 1989), including natural disasters and accidents (e.g., Madakasira & O'Brien, 1987; Wilkinson, 1983), war-related situations (e.g., World War I: Brown, 1918, 1919, 1920-1921; McDougall, 1920-1921; Myers, 1915, 1916; Rivers, 1918; Southard, 1919; Thom & Fenton, 1920; Wingfield, 1920; World War II: Fisher, 1943, 1945; Grinker & Spiegel, 1943, 1945; Henderson & Moore, 1944; Kardiner, 1941; Kardiner & Spiegel, 1947; Kubie, 1943; Parfitt & Carlyle-Gall, 1944; Sargant & Slater, 1941; Simmel, 1944; Torrie, 1944; Tureen & Stein, 1949; Watkins, 1949; and subsequent wars: Archibald & Tuddenham, 1965; Cavenar & Nash, 1976; El-Rayes, 1982; Hendin, Haas, Singer et al., 1984; Kalman, 1977; Kolb, 1985; Perry & Jacobs, 1982; Silver & Kelley, 1985; Sonnenberg, Blank, & Talbott, 1985; D. Spiegel, 1981), kidnapping, rape, burns, torture and concentration camp experiences (e.g., Goldfeld, Mollica, Pesavento, et al., 1988; Jaffe, 1968; Kaszniak et al., 1988; Kinzie, 1993; Krystal, 1993; Niederland, 1968), and physical and sexual abuse (e.g., Agosta & Loring, 1988; Berliner & Wheeler, 1987; Blake-White &

Kline, 1985; Briere & Conte, 1993; Burkett & Bruni, 1993; Feldman-Summers & Pope, 1994; Gelinas, 1983; Herman, 1985; Herman & Schatzow, 1987; Loftus, Polonsky, & Fullilove, 1994; Maltz, 1988; Williams, 1992).

Overall, "memory failure" was a symptom discovered in 34% of patients diagnosed as having post-traumatic stress disorder (Horowitz, Wilner, Kaltreider, & Alvarez, 1980). Bremner, Scott, Delaney, Southwick, Mason, Johnson, Innis, McCarthy, and Charney (1993) documented that Vietnam veterans with PTSD scored significantly lower than matched comparison subjects on measures for immediate and delayed recall, and total recall.

Certainly some of the studies and reports cited above contain imperfections in methodology, as one might naturally expect "because we are in the odd position of asking people about a memory for forgetting a memory" (Loftus et al., 1994, p. 82). For example, in the Briere and Conte (1993) and Williams (1992) studies, questions were asked with some degree of ambiguity that might have resulted in some degree of overreporting of repressed memory. And in Briere and Conte (1993) and Herman and Schatzow (1987) all the subjects were patients in therapy who could have potentially been influenced by therapists. In the latter study, the method of corroboration of the abuse was not reported, which is not ideal. Feldman-Summers and Pope's (1994) results were based on self-reports, and even though 47% of those with delayed recollection of their abuse reported finding some corroboration, this could not be independently confirmed while still assuring anonymity.

On the other hand, the tremendous volume of data available clearly support the existence of traumatic amnesia or robust repression (Spiegel & Scheflin, 1994). The American Psychiatric Association (1994) position statement on memories of sexual abuse also supports the existence of traumatic amnesia. Kenneth Lanning (1994) of the FBI has reported that the existence of robust repression is undeniable based upon FBI recovery of child pornography films where many of the children, when contacted as adults, had no recollection of the abuses which had been documented on film. Thus, the weight of available evidence strongly supports the existence of traumatic amnesia and delayed recall, but what still remains at issue is whether the genuine base rate of repressed memory in an abuse population might be something closer to 19% (Loftus et al., 1994) 38% (Williams, 1992), 40% (FeldmanSummers, 1994), or 59% (Briere & Conte, 1993).

Some persons have argued that mental health patients who are depressed will, because of their depression, negatively distort their memories and may recall nonexistent abuse. However, concerning memory research in general, Singer and Salovey (1988), reviewing the scientific literature on the influence of mood and retrieval of personal memories, reached the conclusion that negative or depressed moods tended to have minimal impact on the recall of memories, whereas a happy mood facilitated the recall of more congruent memories. In comprehensively reviewing the literature on psychopathology and early memory,

Brewin, Andrews, and Gotlib (1993) reached a similar important conclusion that depressed mood *did not* cause a distorting effect in the recall of childhood experiences, and that adult reports of being abused as children should be given as much credence as other reports of childhood experience. They further cited studies indicating that recall by parents tends to be significantly more distorted than the recall of their children. They summarized:

> These data also help to rebut suggestions that depressed individuals report more adverse childhood experiences for motivational reasons, for example, because they wish to justify their current symptoms or to comply with the wishes of their therapist (Lewinsohn & Rosenbaum, 1987; see also Blaney, 1986), or because they have internalized common ideas about links between parenting and psychopathology, which lead them to 'rewrite' their autobiographies to fit in with societal expectations (Gerlsma et al., 1990) (p. 91).... We believe that parents' reports are likely to be particularly unreliable if there has been serious maltreatment such as neglect or emotional, physical, or sexual abuse of their children.... Comparable data from studies of spouse abuse indicate low to moderate agreement between spouses on the incidence of marital violence, with victims reporting more violence than aggressors.... Relative to spousal and independent reports, a high proportion of violent men systematically minimize the frequency and severity of their aggressive actions (Dutton, 1986). Compared with those of other family members, siblings' reports of childhood experiences were found by Schwarz et al. (1985) to be the most valid and the most similar to those of their brothers and sisters. Although the influence of a common family mythology on sibling reports cannot be ruled out, we suggest that the testimony of siblings raised in the same household is preferable to that of parents.... Parental reports appear particularly suspect, and it is probably no accident that critics of retrospective recall such as Halverson (1988) point primarily to studies of parental recall of their children to justify their stance (p. 92).

Memory Retrieval

There is evidence that memories lost through trauma can be accurately retrieved. However, because memory can be malleable, the elicitation of memories must be conducted very carefully in order to maximize accuracy. Numerous non-hypnotic methods have been used in efforts to evoke memories, including general clinical interviews, reinstatement of contextual cues, dream interpretation, free association, and journaling. In clinical interviews, without the use of formal hypnosis, suggestions may be conveyed through leading questions, interviewer expectations and bias, reinforcement of patient productions, and questions focused on material that is difficult to verify. Patients may also enter therapy with potentially contaminating preconceptions about etiologic factors, or with memories that have come from associations with friends, literature, or the media. It is important for the therapist to ascertain what factors may have shaped the patient's ideas about influences from the past or beliefs that abuse may have occurred. Therapists should also be aware that there is empirical literature suggesting that when an examiner presses an individual research subject to provide more information about a past event, a significant number of such participants will produce additional material which may or may not be accurate (Erdelyi, 1985). Thus, because repeated recall trials produce incremental information, some of which is accurate and some of which is inaccurate, the use of hypnosis may sometimes elicit new information simply because it constitutes one more recall trial. But, without external corroboration, memories retrieved in therapy, with or without hypnosis, or indeed memories in general, cannot be assumed to be fully accurate.

SECTION 2

THE CURRENT STATE OF SCIENTIFIC RESEARCH ON HYPNOSIS AND MEMORY

There is general agreement among contemporary cognitive scientists that a subject's recollection of an earlier event can be significantly affected by a variety of non-hypnotic variables, e.g., personal significance of the event, length of time after the event, type of test (i.e., recall vs. recognition) used to assess memory for the event, exposure to different demand characteristics before or during the subject's attempt to remember, being asked leading questions about the event, exposure to misleading information about the event, etc. (Loftus, 1979). Interestingly, most of the published empirical studies which have been reported as demonstrating the deleterious effect of hypnosis on the accuracy of a person's memory also contained one or more kinds of those previously known non-hypnotic influences within some part of the "hypnotic" procedures. This type of methodological shortcoming confounds hypnosis with various nonhypnotic variables which past research has demonstrated to be sufficient to cause memory contamination effects. Consequently, many prior studies which have reported that hypnosis increases inaccurate recollections may have reached a specious conclusion. In fact, a more plausible explanation of these previous investigations is that these non-hypnotic factors (embedded within the hypnotic procedure) may have impaired or altered memory for an earlier event. Whether hypnosis itself was sufficient to produce a similar degree of contamination as these non-hypnotic influences, or significantly increased the size of this effect when used in combination with them, cannot be determined based on the results of such methodologically flawed research. At the same time it must be acknowledged that non-hypnotic influences (e.g., context reinstatement) included with hypnosis may account for positive effects of hypnosis on memory that have been found (Yuille & Kim, 1987). Future studies regarding the effect of hypnotic procedures on memory should avoid confounding hypnosis with known, potent nonhypnotic biasing variables.

The scientific literature, however, does clearly indicate that memory (particularly for details) is imperfect, whether or not formal hypnosis is used. People have been shown to be capable of filling in gaps of memory with confabulated information, of distorting information, and of being influenced in what is "remembered" by leading questions or suggestions. Overall, most academic laboratory studies have found that hypnosis does not generally seem to improve normal memory in normally functioning persons with normal recall ability (Erdelyi, 1988). This research, despite having imperfections and flaws in design, may be reaching relatively accurate conclusions for the particular problem and population studied. The subject matter in this research has primarily consisted of memory for details, briefly observed, that were associated with complex occurrences, thus representing the type of information one would anticipate to be most easily lost to memory.

These findings, however, have led some individuals to overgeneralize inappropriately and question the use of hypnosis with abuse or crime victims. But, as noted earlier, the academic hypnosis and memory research that has been done, as reviewed up until about a decade ago by the AMA Council on Scientific Affairs report (1985), does not provide answers that are in any way definitive about the applications of hypnosis with memory in clinical situations involving abuse, or in forensic cases involving traumatic or highly affect-laden memory. As even the AMA report recognized, "Generalization from the laboratory to the real world depends on the degree to which the laboratory situation accurately represents the field situation" (p. 1920).

There are some serious deficiencies and shortcomings in the existing research (Scheflin, Brown & Hammond, in press; Spiegel, 1980; Spiegel & Spiegel, 1987; Watkins, 1989, 1993) that must prevent scientists from generalizing beyond the population on whom the existing research was performed--normal individuals with normal memory. For example, samples in studies of hypnosis and memory are not random samples of victims of abuse or trauma, or of witnesses to actual crimes, whose memories have been blocked by emotional factors. The relevance of personally experienced trauma and emotion have been ignored in laboratory studies of hypnosis and memory. While trauma may enhance encoding, it may also block retrieval. Subjects in memory and hypnosis studies have been college students, not representative of a population suffering with traumatic blocks to memory, on whom no hypnosis laboratory studies exist. Due to the profound limitations and the completely different population and problem that has been studied, a recent law review article (Kanovitz, 1992) on hypnosis, memory and the law concluded:

> Because the research community has not studied the impact of childhood sexual abuse or any other major traumas on memory or the impact of hypnosis on subjects who have been traumatized, experimentalist testimony about the unreliability of memory may bear little relevance to the trustworthiness of memories restored in psychotherapy (p. 1226).

Another major problem with existing studies failing to find hypermnesia (increased memory accessibility or memory enhancement) is that they have too often used questionable criteria such as nonsense syllables, paired-associate words, faces, slides of objects, numbers, word lists and line drawings. Such criteria are not likely to be associated with negative emotion or to be so affect-laden that they would be blocked from memory, and their lack of personal relevance would not be anticipated to cause the data to imprint itself in someone's mind. Even when videotapes of staged robberies are used, research suggests that this type of stimulus material may not always genuinely produce the same kind of impact on research subject "witnesses" as it does upon real witnesses (Christianson & Hubinette, 1993; Cutshall & Yuille, 1989; Fisher, Geiselman, & Amador, 1989; Yuille & Cutshall, 1986; Yuille & Kim, 1987).

However, it has been discovered that the closer the research design is to real life uses of hypnosis, the more likely hypnosis facilitates memory without increase in errors (Geiselman & Machlovitz, 1987). Geiselman et al. (1985) found that hypnosis interviews by experienced persons produced 35% more correct facts than standard police interviews, and Geiselman and Machlovitz (1987) concluded that while it is conceivable that a hypnotist could be ineffective or cause confabulation, their analysis of 38 experiments did not support this claim and the differences in experimental methodology were what predicted the success or failure of hypnosis aided recall. "Rather, hypnosis memory recall was most likely to be successful when more natural conditions obtained" (p. 45). Relatedly, researchers who take the position that hypnotically retrieved memories are likely to be distorted and who, therefore, insist that all forensic interviews must be fully videotaped to evaluate potential contamination, have not applied these same strict criteria to their own hypnotic and pre- and post-hypnotic work with research subjects. Thus, they fail to control for the potential contamination that their own skeptical viewpoints have on experimental outcomes (Watkins, 1993). In many instances, the specific, detailed suggestions given to subjects are not even provided to allow further scientific scrutiny for potential experimental bias.

Erdelyi (1994) concluded that hypermnesia or enhanced memory exists and "occurs with or without hypnosis," but he believes that "hypnosis does not uniquely add to (or subtract from) hypermnesia" (p. 386) with non-traumatic memory. He believes that simply repeated retrieval efforts (whether in hypnosis or not) are what is responsible for increased recall. Thus, for example, Geiselman et al. (1985) found a nonhypnotic guided memory interview (which took twice the time and used three times as many questions as hypnosis) increased correct recall as much as a hypnotic procedure (and both yielded more than a police interview). But, the fact remains that the repeated retrieval effort was more effective in enhancing recall, whether it was conducted with or without hypnosis. Even if this conclusion of equivalency were found to hold for traumatic memory as well (which it may not), why should one's preference for one or the other technique matter? Academicians with theoretical interests may be concerned with what aspect of a procedure is effective in enhancing non-traumatic memory recall, but whether that variable is embedded within a hypnotic procedure, or a much longer "cognitive interview" is irrelevant in actual life circumstances, as long as it produces hypermnesia.

Relatedly, several extensive reviews of literature on memory and hypnosis (Kanovitz, 1992; Relinger, 1984; Scheflin & Shapiro, 1989; Scheflin, Brown & Hammond, in press; Smith, 1983; Weitzenhoffer, 1953) all reached the conclusion that although hypnosis does not aid in the recall of meaningless stimuli, it may facilitate recall of personally meaningful information or material associated with emotional situations. This conclusion was also reached by White, Fox, and Harris in 1940, citing that the type of stimulus used by a hypnosis researcher would determine the nature of recall--yet, research using such meaningless stimuli continued into the 1960's, 1970's, 1980's, and even the 1990's!

We believe that clinically relevant research is needed. Frankel (1988, p. 250) expressed similar perceptions and suggested that narrow laboratory studies "might best be regarded as beacons, not barriers. Part of their purpose is to illuminate, not to dictate, the paths that we follow clinically (p. 263). McConkey's (1992) review of this literature concluded that, "The varying findings [about hypnosis and memory] that have been reported in the literature appear to have as much to do with the experimental methods used as they do with the phenomena being investigated. This is an important point to underscore" (p. 411).

Problems like those cited above have plagued eyewitness memory research in general, even apart from hypnosis (e.g., Zaragoza & Koshmidir, 1989). There was such a consistent pattern of reliable differences between laboratory results of memory with uninvolved bystander witnesses and the witness of real-life emotional events, that these types of results led Fisher et al. (1989) to conclude: "If this difference between laboratory and field studies continues to appear, one may question the validity of describing in court the accuracy rates found in the laboratory as evidence of the general unreliability of eyewitness testimony in field cases" (p. 725). However, Christianson (1992d) notes that recent real life studies and simulation studies of memory for emotional events are consistent in finding that centrally important information is better retained and less likely to be forgotten. Christianson and Hubinette (1993) pointed out that the discrepancy in studies in many instances seems due to what certain researchers concentrate on in their studies, with the incongruence often due to differences in the type of memory test, time of test, and type of detail examined. Thus certain researchers examine accuracy and persistence of memory (e.g., Christianson, 1984; Heuer & Reisberg, 1990; Reisberg, Heuer, McLean, & O'Shaughnessy, 1988; Yuille & Cutshall, 1986), while other investigators focus on errors in memory and deterioration of memory over time (e.g., Clifford & Hollin, 1981; Clifford & Scott, 1978; Loftus & Burns, 1982; Neisser & Harsch, 1990; Wagenaar & Groeneweg, 1990).

The laboratory literature on hypnosis and memory is also characterized by another major flaw: it fails to distinguish between the global concept of hypnosis and the many techniques, types of suggestions, and ways hypnosis may be used. This is similar to the failing that has been commonplace for many years throughout the general psychotherapy research literature of only discussing the effectiveness of "psychotherapy" or "hypnotic treatments," without explicating the specific methods, individual suggestions, and techniques used in each study of "psychotherapy" or "hypnosis."

Inasmuch as studies and real world cases do seem to suggest that hypnotic efforts do improve recall under some conditions for some individuals (e.g., Block, 1976; Kaszniak, et al., 1988; Kroger & Douce, 1979; Raginsky, 1969), investigations with improved ecological validity should address why and when memory may be enhanced. Furthermore, instead of only pursuing a one-sided research orientation of evaluating the fallibility of memory for details, balanced research is needed that also examines the relative overall accuracy of recall of highly emotion-laden memories. Since hypnosis is believed by many people in the field to be a controlled dissociation (e.g., Hilgard, 1977, 1986; Spiegel, 1993; Spiegel & Greenleaf, 1992), and because of the evidence that many trauma and abuse victims enter trance-like, dissociative states during and after trauma (e.g., Eth & Pynoos, 1985; Krystal, 1993; Terr, 1991), recreating an emotional and dissociative context through hypnosis integrated within psychotherapy may facilitate both the recovery and working through of traumatic memories (Spiegel, 1993).

Thus, for example, Kroger and Douce (1979) cited the real world example of a kidnapping and rape where a teenaged victim was hypnotized and remembered considerable additional details. She recalled unique rust spots on the car, articles inside the car, a specific detail about a gear shift knob, a noise made by a window when rolled up, a service station location, a physical description of a credit card used, and what a gas station repairman said needed fixing on the car. These hypnotically obtained details were all independently confirmed, and the suspect was located. Subsequently, other young girls that the man had sexually abused came forward, and he was convicted. Block (1976) similarly describes the successful role of hypnosis in numerous major criminal cases and in a variety of cases reported by the Israeli National Police Force.

Hypnosis may particularly aid in the recall of meaningful, affect-laden events, for example, in situations where emotional trauma has created a block to memory, because of the state-dependent nature of some memories and the manner in which the encoding context and mood may be reinstated through hypnosis. Hypnosis may also facilitate memory recall in situations where early traumatic memories were encoded in visual images more than in verbal form (Terr, 1988) because hypnosis enhances the vividness of imagery and imagery is greater in persons responsive to hypnosis (e.g., Bowers, 1976; Crawford & Allen, 1983; Sanders, 1969; Sheehan, 1979; Spanos, Brett, Menary & Cross, 1987). In addition, entirely apart from memory recall, hypnotic reframing and reinterpretation, ego-strengthening, and suggestions for symptom management are perceived as being of particular therapeutic value in reducing symptoms that interfere with memory performance and ultimately in the working through of trauma.

Hypnosis is not magical in facilitating hypermnesia, but with emotion-laden memories for meaningful material, we believe it likely that hypnosis has the potential to clearly prove helpful with some individuals. Memory is not entirely accurate no matter what method is used to examine the past, and it may be influenced by waking or hypnotic suggestions. But, as a recent law review article concluded, "Psychodynamic psychotherapies use techniques to uncover the past that are slower than hypnosis and provide no superior guarantee that memories recovered are accurate", "'talking' psychotherapies are as capable of implanting false memories of childhood sexual abuse as hypnotic ones," and "there is as much opportunity for memory alteration to occur in nonhypnotic psychotherapies as in hypnotic ones" (pp. 1243, 1246, & 1251) (Kanovitz, 1992).

Apart from the accuracy of memory, research has shown that an increase in false feelings of confidence may and often does occur when hypnosis is used to elicit memories in highly hypnotizable persons (e.g., Dywan & Bowers, 1983; Laurence, 1982; Laurence & Perry, 1983; Rainer, 1983; Sheehan & Grigg, 1985; Sheehan, Grigg & McCann, 1984; Zelig & Beidleman, 1981), but this is not the case in all studies (e.g., Mingay, 1986; Putnam, 1979; Sanders & Simons, 1983; Spanos et al., 1989; Yuille & McEwan, 1985; Zelig & Beidleman, 1981). From examining the nature of suggestions used in studies with findings of increased confidence (when they were included in reports), we believe that when enhanced confidence does occur it may well be due to the nature of the specific suggestions given and the influence of social psychological variables (e.g., that create expectations on the part of the subject for accurate recall), rather than hypnosis itself. For example, Sheehan et al. (1991) "emphasized to subjects that everything that had happened in the video had been recorded in their minds" and "that they may remember events and details that their conscious mind had forgotten but that their subconscious mind would remember" (p. 132).

In other words, it may well be the specific hypnotic technique, suggestions, and prehypnotic expectations concerning the nature of hypnosis that may result in increased confidence, and not simply the fact that hypnosis was used. Subject beliefs prior to hypnosis have been shown to impact the nature of hypnotic experiences (e.g., Baker, 1982; Council et al., 1983; Council et al., 1986; Kirsch, 1991; Kirsch et al., 1987; Johnston et al., 1989; Spanos et al., 1991; Wickless & Kirsch, 1989). Despite our belief that hypnotic response is influenced by more than only the subject's expectations, it is clear that patient beliefs and expectations have a definite impact on patient productions that should be considered, and may be influenced by waking suggestions from therapists.

Concerning a patient's expectations, previous studies have shown that hypnosis has been publicly misperceived by many people as facilitating vivid reinstatement of memories (McConkey & Jupp, 1985; McConkey, Roche, & Sheehan, 1989; Wilson, Greene, & Loftus, 1986), which might cause a jury to give added weight to recollections obtained through hypnosis (Diamond, 1980; Odgers, 1988). Nonetheless, juries (and patients) may be educated to create neutral expectations about hypnosis. Furthermore, given the recent publicity about false memories of child abuse (which have often presented hypnosis in a strongly negative light), there is a need to repeat earlier studies about public conceptions of hypnosis. Patient expectations about hypnosis may be evaluated pre-hypnotically, and efforts made to create realistic and neutral expectations.

Hypnosis, Nonhypnosis and Pseudomemories

Memories may be contaminated and pseudomemories created as a result of uncontrolled social psychological variables and situational demands (Lynn, Rhue, Myers, & Weekes, 1994; McCloskey & Zaragoza, 1985; Murrey, Cross, & Whipple, 1992, 1992; Zaragoza & Koshmidir, 1989). A brief introduction is in order on the competing theoretical explanations of non-hypnotic memory contamination and pseudomemory production. While there is broad consensus that numerous types of nonhypnotic factors can significantly effect the accuracy of a persons' recollection for past events in controlled laboratory contexts, no one conceptual account regarding the mechanism(s) underlying these effects has achieved wide scientific acceptance. Four competing theories have received the most attention. The major difference between these four conceptual accounts concerns whether a persons' recollection for the original stimulus detail is assumed to be no longer available in their memory store or whether it is regarded as being potentially available, but not readily accessible (i.e., Tulving & Pearlstone, 1966).

The Memory Alteration Hypothesis. The memory alteration hypothesis (MAH) characterizes memory as a dynamic process that is continuously being updated so that one's earliest memory traces are constantly being altered over time. Exposure to postevent information is one way of causing such changes in a person's previous memory traces. The MAH proposes that after such trace transformations have taken place, it is no longer possible for the person to access prior memories because they have been permanently overwritten (Loftus, 1979).

The Memory Coexistence Hypothesis. The memory coexistence hypothesis (MCH) proposes that exposure to postevent information coexists with the earlier memory and that both are available (Bekerian & Bowers, 1983; Bowers & Bekerian, 1984; Christiaansen & Ochalek, 1983). However, different stimulus factors (e.g., recency effects, serial order effects, contextual reinstatement effects, postevent information credibility discounting effects) can effect a subject's final memory test performance during testing because they render the memory for postevent information more accessible than the original memory. Experimental manipulations have been found to be able to reverse this, however, making the original memory more accessible.

The Demand Characteristics Hypothesis. The demand characteristics hypothesis (DCH) proposes that many research subjects figure out the experimenters' hypothesis and perceive a strong social demand to comply with it. Hence, such subjects deliberately alter their performance on a memory test to acquiesce to this perceived social demand to help the experimenters prove their theory by responding in the expected manner (Weinberg, Wadsworth, & Baron, 1983).

The Response Bias Hypothesis. The response bias hypothesis (RBH) proposes that memory changes may represent methodological artifacts (e.g., McCloskey & Zaragoza, 1985; Zaragoza & Koshmidir, 1989). Proponents of RBH have empirically demonstrated that exposure to inaccurate postevent information does not effect final memory test performance if the target items do not contain response options which correspond to the inaccurate postevent information. Based on this kind of evidence, McCloskey and Zaragoza (1985) argued that if postevent information exposure actually overwrote a persons' initially accurate memory, then they should guess between the original detail and a new inaccurate detail with a 50% chance rate of choosing the correct answer. However, 70% or more of subjects given such a final memory test selected the original detail. Unfortunately, other interpretations of this finding consistent with MAH are plausible.

Hypnosis and Pseudomemory. The data that hypnosis may create false memories stems mostly from laboratory-based research on student samples who score high or moderately high in hypnotic responsivity (e.g. Barnier & McConkey, 1992; Labelle, Laurence, Nadon, & Perry, 1990; McConkey, Labelle, Bibb, & Bryant, 1990; Sheehan, Statham, & Jamieson, 1991a,b). The lower a person scores in hypnotizability, the less vulnerable he or she appears to be for accepting suggestions for pseudomemories, but high and moderately hypnotizable persons are more vulnerable to suggestions for pseudomemories than low hypnotizable subjects. However, in this research, often only a minority of subjects produce false memories, and these are generally with regard to peripheral details. These results demonstrate simply that in a selected portion of the population it *may sometimes* be possible to create a false memory report for detail. Furthermore, giving hypnotic suggestions for age regression and to re-experience an event have not been found to be the variables associated with the creation of pseudomemories (Lynn, Milano, & Weekes, 1991).

Hypnosis itself does not appear to be a significant biasing factor in the creation of pseudomemories, contributing relatively little to the overall variance of pseudomemory production. As McConkey (1992) concluded: "There may not be anything particularly hypnotic about hypnotic pseudomemory" (p. 423), and "it is wrong to assume that variation in memory is necessarily a function of hypnotic procedures" (p. 424). Research demonstrates that reports of pseudomemories may be created through suggestion without hypnosis (Garry & Loftus, 1994; Loftus & Coan, in press) as well as in hypnosis, and social influence appears to be the primary factor contributing to their production. Brown (1995) concluded that hypnotizability was the primary risk factor, rather than the use of hypnosis, and that social factors contributed at least as much if not more than hypnotizability level to the production of pseudomemories. He further indicated:

> Moreover, false beliefs in psychotherapy are very likely to occur when an *interaction of four primary risk factors* are present: 1) hypnotizability; 2) uncertainty about past events; 3) clear evidence

of interrogatory suggestive influence; and 4) extratherapeutic social influences, e.g., peer and familial influences, especially self help group experiences, and available socio-cultural beliefs.

Along with social influence, the quality of higher hypnotizability within a patient (not hypnosis) appears to be implicated (Barnier & McConkey, 1992; Labelle, et al., 1990; McConkey, et al., 1990; Sheehan, Garnett, & Robertson, 1993; Sheehan et al., 1991a,b). Thus, for example, Sheehan et al. (1993) found that highly hypnotizable persons *in hypnosis* were not more vulnerable to the effects of leading questions than high hypnotizable persons not in hypnosis.

The use of leading questions in nonhypnotic situations has been shown in a number of empirical studies to significantly influence how people describe recollections of past events (summarized in Loftus, 1979). Any question can be characterized as "leading" if either its form or content suggests to the person what answer is desired or leads him or her to the desired answer. For example, Loftus and Palmer (1974) showed a group of college students a film about an automobile accident. Later, some subjects were asked to estimate "how fast were the cars going when they *smashed* each other?" In contrast, other subjects were queried about "how fast were the cars going when they *contacted* each other?" Their results showed that subjects asked the question containing the word "smashed" gave a significantly higher speed estimate (40.8 mph) than those asked the same question with the word "contacted" (30.8 mph). Although the words in both questions referred to the coming together of two objects, each differed in what they implied about the speed and force of impact. However, it should also be noted that the one attempt to replicate this study in a "real world" context discovered that all the subjects resisted such suggestions (Yuille & Cutshall, 1986). Yuille (1994) has interpreted this difference by suggesting that the context (e.g., experimental versus real life) may influence the degree to which a person is susceptible to leading questions. As Yuille (1994) further reports, "I am not suggesting that leading questions are not a problem, clearly they are. However, context may effect the degree to which an individual is susceptible to particular leading questions." It should be noted that the literature of leading questions has not been scientifically studied with enough emphasis on varying contexts. While all researchers would likely agree that leading questions can influence memory, the literature of leading questions does not yet permit a full context analysis.

Another common type of leading question is one which contains the article "the" instead of "a" (Loftus & Zanni, 1975). For example, asking a witness, "Did you see *the* stop sign," is not the same as asking, "Did you see *a* stop sign?" The former question suggests the existence of a stop sign while the latter query does not contain such an implication. A more neutral question would be, "Tell me what comes to you, if anything?" Thus, there is evidence that indirect suggestions such as implications (Hammond, 1990) may be influential in nonhypnotic as well as hypnotic states. Because of such findings, we believe clinicians must err on the side of cautiousness and minimize such questions with regard to memory recall in any type of clinical interaction, even though one must be cautious about generalizing from such misinformation studies about peripheral details in laboratory contexts to real life recollections of actual, personally experienced events such as trauma.

Persons appear more vulnerable to creating a pseudomemory if they hold definite and congruent personal beliefs (e.g., in reincarnation) prior to hypnosis, and are expecting to find something compatible with this belief (e.g., an event in a past life) (Baker, 1982; Spanos et al., 1991a) which is not verifiable (Lynn, Milano, & Weekes, 1992; Lynn, Weekes & Milano, 1989; McCann & Sheehan, 1987, 1988) and has a high perceived likelihood of occurrence (Weekes, Lynn & Myers, 1993). We suspect that a large proportion of patients who do not already recall abuse, probably would not consider abuse as something that would have a high likelihood of having occurred unless they came from a generally abusive background. (To provide objectivity, during routine patient evaluations, clinicians can ask patients who do not recall abuse to rate their belief in the likelihood that they were abused but do not recall it.) However, it must be considered possible that this expectation could be altered by a therapist's confident expression of a hypothesis that sexual abuse likely accounted for the patient's symptoms and could have been repressed. Thus, therapists should be cautious about sharing such hypotheses that could potentially alter a patient's expectancies. To avoid errors of overconfidence, therapists likewise should not create an expectancy that everything is recorded in the patient's mind and that hypnosis will uncover whatever is there.

However, in the research it actually appears that in many cases pseudomemory effects represent something more akin to a response bias resulting from uncontrolled social psychological variables and situational demands, rather than representing a genuine distortion or change of memory, (Lynn et al., 1994; McCloskey & Zaragoza, 1985; Murrey et al., 1992; Zaragoza & Koshmidir, 1989). As the work of Sheehan and McConkey (1982) on the EAT (experiential analysis technique) demonstrate, hypnotic subjects retain the ability to monitor external events as they process suggestions, and remain responsive to the demand characteristics of experimenters and try to please experimenters (Lynn et al., 1989; McCann & Sheehan, 1987, 1988, 1989). Laboratory research finds that the majority of people in hypnosis, including even high hypnotizable subjects, do not mistake hypnotically suggested fantasies for actual events. Rather, several studies indicate that when subjects are motivated to give unbiased, honest reports, pseudomemory reports appear to be minimized (e.g., Lynn et al., 1989; Murrey et al., 1992; Spanos et al., 1989), just as they are when the person is questioned away from the compliance pressure of the experimental testing context (e.g., McConkey et al., 1990). There is also evidence that hypnotic pseudomemory can be breached by exposure to evidence relating to the original events (e.g., McCann & Sheehan, 1987, 1989), and is low when the target of the pseudomemory suggestion is publicly verifiable (Lynn, Milano, & Weekes, 1992; McCann & Sheehan, 1987,

1988). Furthermore, the rate of pseudomemory production in high hypnotizable persons varies dramatically in studies (from 80% to 0%!), depending on the nature of the testing circumstances, of the suggested pseudomemory, and the demand characteristics of the experiment.

At least four other reasons to limit generalization from laboratory research to real life situations should be mentioned. Some studies use exceedingly liberal criteria for the presence of pseudomemory, such as simply expressing confusion or uncertainty (e.g., Labelle et al., 1990; Laurence & Perry, 1983). Barnier and McConkey (1992) believe such criteria may artificially inflate pseudomemory for detail estimates, when in reality their criteria "hardly [represent] a major change in memory," and could be equally interpretable as the absence of pseudomemories. Another problem that plagues the pseudomemory research is the irrelevancy and commonplace nature of many of the implanted memories--something very different from traumatic memory. For example, suggested events include a telephone ringing, pencils dropping, or hearing a noise while asleep in the night. These are innocuous, everyday events tremendously at variance from the real world memories reported by patients.

Another flaw in pseudomemory research is that a number of studies have tested subjects for having a pseudomemory *during* hypnosis, instead of after hypnosis. If a subject complies or reports such a belief during hypnosis, he or she may well feel pressure to continue to give the same consistent response and maintain a consistent role (Leippe, 1980; McCann & Sheehan, 1989; Spanos & McLean, 1986). Furthermore, the data suggest that original memories are not irretrievably lost when a pseudomemory is created through suggestion, and that these distortions are not irreversibly integrated with original memories (McCann & Sheehan, 1988; Murrey et al., 1992).

Finally, it must be pointed out that for ethical reasons experimental hypnotic studies have not sought to emulate reality by creating memories of traumatic events. The only exception is studies by Reyher (e.g., Sommerschield & Reyher, 1973) on induced conflicts, motivations and desires. These studies provide some support for the phenomenon of repression, but were not studies of the pseudomemory phenomenon that controlled for demand characteristics by using a waking suggestion group of high hypnotizables, blinding the hypnotist to the group assignment, and using someone different than the experimenter in a different context to evaluate the ability of subjects to distinguish suggested pseudomemories from reality. Sheehan (1969) concluded that the demand characteristics of the research are responsible for the psychopathology seen in Reyher studies. And, in fact, Smyth (1982), who participated in studies with Reyher, expressed the belief that high hypnotizable subjects "probably become *temporarily* absorbed in the conflictual paramnesias to the point where the suggested fantasies take on an air of reality" (p. 556, emphasis added), and that the resulting emotion combined with desires to fulfill the role of a good hypnotic subject produced the behavior desired in the experiment.

The possibility that corruption of memory by hypnosis would be compounded by increased confidence instilled through hypnosis has been of concern, but as indicated above, when it does occur it may well represent the effects of specific, biasing pre-hypnotic and hypnotic suggestions. Furthermore, hypnotic techniques do not appear to immunize subjects (as suggested by Orne, 1979, and Diamond, 1980) against the effects of cross-examination (e.g., Spanos et al., 1989; Spanos et al., 1991b). Even the Supreme Court has questioned such beliefs. In Rock v. Arkansas (1987) they stated that it "has not been shown that hypnotically enhanced testimony is always so untrustworthy and so immune to the traditional means of evaluating credibility that it should disable a defendant from presenting her version of the events for which she is on trial."

The entire areas of memory, and hypnosis and memory, are complex and both academic researchers and clinicians must admit that there is still a great deal to be learned. One thing seems clear, however, repressed memory exists, and false beliefs about the past also exist, and the reality of one does not preclude the existence of the other (Nash, 1994). Much more clinically relevant research is critically needed, but while we await such research it is *vitally* important for clinicians to work *cautiously* and judiciously with memories of abuse. We are convinced that persons may be led through suggestive interviewing and interrogation techniques, without formal hypnosis. We are equally convinced that hypnosis may be used by a poorly trained clinician in ways that can distort the memory of hypnotized persons.

At various times the literature on hypnosis has demonstrated polar opposite positions. On the one hand, some authors have argued that hypnosis always contaminates memory and, in effect, tampers with the evidence. On the other side of the scale, authors have concluded that hypnosis has a miraculous capacity to cause accurate memories to be reproduced precisely as the events occurred. Courts have relied on both positions, and thereby reached erroneous conclusions. The real question is whether hypnosis, properly used, is any more likely to contaminate memory than the ordinary processes recognized in eyewitness testimony, interrogative questioning, interviewing, or other aspects of suggestion already recognized by courts. McConkey (1992) concluded: "Analyses of the experimental findings on hypnosis and memory have more often than not ended in dire warnings about the negative effects or in proselytizing claims about the positive effects of hypnosis on memory. Overstatement of either kind is not a reasonable conclusion, however" p. 425).

Based on the scientific evidence from numerous studies, this panel concludes that contaminating effects on memory are no more likely to occur from the use of hypnosis than from many nonhypnotic interviewing and interrogative procedures. Therefore, legal rules that single out hypnosis for restrictive treatment are unwarranted. Hypnosis should be treated by the law as any other form of suggestion is treated by the law (Scheflin, 1994a, 1994b; U.S. v Adams; U.S. v Wade).

The committee wishes to emphasize that we believe there is reason to question whether hypnosis itself is innately distorting. We believe that for the most part it is the manner in which hypnosis is sometimes used in eliciting recall of memories and the nature of the subject being hypnotized that contributes to distortion (e.g., Sheehan et al., 1993). We have reviewed many carefully controlled studies suggesting that the same distortions of memory may be produced nonhypnotically as may be produced hypnotically. One of the few outcomes about hypnosis that appears with some consistency that may suggest something unique is the finding that hypnosis may encourage a greater subject confidence in what is recalled. However, as stated earlier, this may well be due to effects of inappropriately biasing waking and hypnotic suggestions that may have created subject expectancies for highly accurate recall that would then instill greater confidence. Further research is needed to adequately evaluate this. Thus, with the possible exception of issues of confidence, we conclude that expectancies created through waking suggestion, unrealistic expectations held by the subject, and leading questions, may clearly add distortion, inaccuracy, and inappropriate confidence in memories, especially with highly hypnotizable persons – *whether they are hypnotized or not.*

The committee has sought to evaluate current scientific knowledge concerning memory, influence, and hypnosis and memory, in a balanced manner. Subsequently, in the interests of encouraging the highest standards of professional practice, we offer the following recommendations to clinicians working with hypnotic age regression and the elicitation of memories.

SECTION 3

A.S.C.H. RECOMMENDATIONS FOR CLINICIANS WORKING WITH HYPNOSIS AND MEMORY WITH PATIENTS WHO MAY HAVE BEEN ABUSED

In Sections 3 and 4, and the appendices that follow, the American Society of Clinical Hypnosis Ad Hoc Committee on Hypnosis and Memory offers recommendations for clinicians working with memory and in the area of forensic hypnosis. The following recommendations describe a range of generally accepted approaches for clinicians who use hypnosis for exploration and for uncovering or the working through of problematic memories of patients. These recommendations attempt to define principles of practice that should generally meet the needs of most patients in most circumstances. However, these recommendations should not be construed as rules, but as suggested guidelines, nor should they be deemed inclusive of all proper methods or exclusive of other methods reasonably directed at obtaining the appropriate results. It is anticipated that it will be necessary to approach some patients' needs in different ways. The ultimate judgment regarding the care of a particular patient must be made by the therapist in light of all of the circumstances presented by the patient, the options available, and available resources. These recommendations are not to be construed as a legal document nor used in a court of law as a standard, because standards of care are determined on the basis of all the facts or circumstances involved in an individual case and are subject to change as scientific knowledge and technology advance and as practice patterns evolve. But, these recommendations are based on a consensus of the committee concerning the status of the scientific literature at the time of publication.

1. Evaluating the Patient

Assessment should be conducted, somatic complaints medically evaluated, and a diagnostic impression established prior to hypnosis. Interviewing concerning historical events should be conducted in a neutral, nonleading manner and the patient's expectancies, goals and perceptions of hypnosis should be explored. If the patient has beliefs that abuse may have occurred, carefully evaluate how the patient came to hold these beliefs. Referral source expectations and their potential contaminating influences should also be considered.

In patients who recall memories of abuse or believe they may have been abused, determine whether they have done any reading, viewed films, attended classes or groups, or associated with persons who have reported similar abuse which may have provided a contaminating influence that the therapist must be cautious not to reinforce. Although such experiences may provide possible contamination that must be considered, we must at the same time objectively consider the possibility that events such as viewing a television program may also simply have provided a contextual cue eliciting a valid memory.

2. Qualifications

Hypnotic age regression and uncovering should only be used by licensed health and mental health professionals with advanced degrees, within their area of expertise. Unlicensed persons using these techniques with potentially traumatic material should be considered as improperly practicing psychotherapy. Prior to using these procedures, licensed professionals should have received thorough training in hypnosis, meeting at least the minimum standards set forth in the A.S.C.H. Standards of Training in Clinical Hypnosis (Hammond & Elkins, 1994) for certification, or similar standards in other countries.

Therapists should study the literature on memory (e.g., Christianson, 1992b, 1992c; Freyd, 1994; Loftus, 1993; Terr, 1988, 1991; van der Kolk & Saporta, 1993; van der Kolk & van der Hart, 1991), and memory and hypnosis (e.g., McConkey, 1992; Pettinati, 1988; Scheflin, Brown, & Hammond, in press), to overcome misunderstandings that may be inadvertently passed on to patients (e.g., that memory is like a tape recorder). Because some memory researchers have polarized around political issues, the grand theory that would harmonize both strands of research has not yet been constructed. Therapists must, therefore, realize and take into account the emphasis and limitations of various memory researchers, so that they can adopt a balanced point of view. For example, some researchers (e.g., Laurence, Loftus, Orne, Perry, Spanos) have generally focused on normal, not traumatic memory, and on inaccuracy, distortion, and decline in memory. Other researchers have focused more on emotional, real life, and traumatic memory, as well as on accuracy or persistence of memory (e.g., Christianson, Geiselman, Heuer, LeDoux, Reisberg, Terr, Yuille, van der Kolk). Clinicians must appreciate that although traumatic memories might ofttimes have relative overall accuracy, memory is also somewhat malleable and therapeutic work must proceed in a manner that avoids undue influence.

Hypnotic uncovering techniques should only be used by health professionals with systematic training in hypnosis (Hammond & Elkins, 1994), and who in addition have psychotherapeutic training in working with victims of abuse or trauma. Therapists using hypnosis, even in purely clinical contexts, may also wish to consult with legal counsel concerning the most current legal rulings in their jurisdiction regarding the admissibility of hypnotically refreshed recollection.

3. Preconditions for Hypnotic Uncovering and the Importance of Informed Consent

Within a psychotherapeutic context, what are the conditions in which more exploratory hypnotic techniques (Brown & Fromm, 1986; Rossi & Cheek, 1988; Watkins, 1992) (used to encourage insight into intrapersonal dynamics, adaptive functions or the contribution of feelings or earlier life experiences to current problems) seem more appropriate or indicated, as contrasted with the use of suggestive hypnosis (Hammond, 1990, 1994) which focuses on offering suggestions for symptom amelioration or management? When patients present with long-standing and complex symptoms that have generalized to a larger number of life areas, where the initial assessment suggests adaptive functions and conflicts may be associated with patient problems, and where the patient's present life stressors and relationships do not seem to adequately account for symptomatic complaints, insight-oriented hypnotic techniques seem reasonably indicated as part of treatment. Hypnotic uncovering also seems most compatible with patients possessing adequate impulse control and ability to tolerate affect involved in exploration, who are psychologically-minded, verbal, intelligent and who have capacity for insight, and in patients who enter treatment with the expectation that insight will be curative and who wish to pursue a therapeutic goal of self-awareness. An insight-oriented hypnotic approach to explore resistance may also be indicated when, in a patient who is responsive to hypnosis, several sessions of suggestive therapy have not produced encouraging symptomatic improvement.

It is recommended that age regression should not be done with a patient who does not give permission for the procedure. In more severely disturbed patients (e.g. with serious borderline conditions, psychosis), therapists should not use hypnosis for age regression or exploration, as contrasted with using hypnosis for symptom management and ego-strengthening. When a patient demonstrates an inability to organize material, displays extreme emotional lability, fragile ego-strength, or is already having spontaneous abreactions and frequent dissociative episodes, hypnotic uncovering techniques that loosen already tenuous control should generally be delayed until further stabilization has occurred. When these techniques are used with such patients they should be used with caution and only by experienced hypnotherapists. These hypnotic methods should also be used with discretion in medically impaired patients for whom the strain of recalling potentially traumatic material may pose dangers to physical health. Furthermore, therapists should be cautious about distortions to which more seriously disturbed patients may be prone by the nature of their particular disorders, but should also realize that psychiatric disturbance does not necessarily compromise the validity or reliability of patient memories (Brewin, Andrews, & Gotlib, 1993). Finally, in the event that issues arise in the therapy with legal ramifications, it is recommended that the therapist should consult legal counsel.

In contrast to insight-oriented techniques, a more parsimonious, short-term suggestive approach to hypnosis will more often be the initial treatment of choice in treating less complex clinical conditions, such as habit disorders, medical conditions, and monosymptomatic or situational problems. Tentative selection criteria for brief suggestive hypnosis may include patients with a history of relatively adequate functioning and adjustment prior to the current problem, who have symptoms that are perceived as ego-dystonic, good motivation to make changes, and who have focal problems that are circumscribed and specific. Suggestive hypnosis also seems most appropriate with patients with problems of more recent origin and onset, who have the capacity to follow-through with homework (e.g., self-hypnosis), and who are capable of establishing an unambivalent and positive therapeutic alliance and display a willingness to cooperate and capacity to trust the therapist. Under such conditions, when 2-4 sessions of suggestive hypnosis in a hypnotically responsive patient do not seem to produce encouraging changes, it is reasonable for a therapist to explore the reasons for the resistance and to shift to a more insight-oriented hypnotic strategy.

However, whether the choice is to recommend suggestive hypnosis or insight-oriented hypnotic techniques to the patient, the therapist would be well advised to obtain an informed consent, except in unusual circumstances, such as in a medical crisis in an emergency room. This informed consent should include information designed to protect the rights of patients to testify in court and informing them of the possible limitation of their rights if hypnosis is performed. Furthermore, such techniques should generally be used with patients after there has been a discussion about the issue that memory is imperfect, concerning hypnosis and memory, and until efforts have been made to structure realistic and neutral expectations concerning the elicitation of further material and its potential accuracy. The therapist should be aware that hypnosis is not a truth serum or like the public image of a polygraph (which has likewise been found to be imperfect and is nonadmissable in court)--patients may lie, confabulate, or fantasize in hypnosis, and this should be conveyed to the patient as part of education concerning myths about hypnosis.

4. Creating Neutral Expectations Concerning the Production of New or Accurate Memories.

When increased confidence in memories occurs following hypnosis, it is most likely due to the use of suggestions that create expectations on the part of the patient for accurate recall. Such suggestions may be given prior to and during hypnosis, and in fact, are often part of traditional hypnotic work. There is an appropriate time and place for a therapist to confidently engender expectancies that the patient will get better. Age regression, however, is not the time to utilize the traditional hypnotic suggestions designed to increase responsiveness.

For example, if a hypnotherapist suggests that the patient's "memory will now increase," that "everything has been recorded in your mind, nothing has been forgotten, and it will now be freely accessible and you can and will clearly remember everything," this will be anticipated to potentially increase both the volume of information produced and patient confidence in what is "remembered." The committee believes such contaminating effects may be controlled considerably when neutral expectations are created prior to hypnosis and during hypnotic induction and age regression. This neutrality should structure patient expectations to the effect that further information may or may not be forthcoming, and may or may not be accurate. Through such measures, errors of increased confidence are more likely to be minimized or eliminated. When a therapist suggests, "You can and will recall everything," patients are given a motivated authorization to guess.

Therapists who have themselves been victims of abuse should exercise particular caution to ensure that their own abuse issues have been adequately resolved. Such individuals should take extra care to monitor their own countertransference reactions and expectations that may be conveyed while providing psychotherapy and hypnosis services.

5. Evaluating Hypnotic Responsivity

It is recommended in working with potential victims of abuse that therapists evaluate hypnotic responsivity, even when the therapist is not necessarily anticipating the therapeutic use of hypnosis. In this regard, it may be advisable for clinicians to consider obtaining a formal measure of hypnotic responsivity (e.g., the Stanford Hypnotic Clinical Scale, the Stanford Hypnotic Susceptibility Scale, Form C, or the Harvard Group Scale of Hypnotic Susceptibility; [see Hilgard & Hilgard, 1983; Weitzenhoffer & Hilgard, 1962; Shor & Orne, 1962] and the Hypnotic Induction Profile [see Spiegel & Spiegel, 1978/1987]) to document the level of hypnotizability and determine the likelihood that the person was actually hypnotized. At a minimum, therapists should elicit hypnotic phenomena of known difficulty level to ascertain hypnotic capacity.

The benefits of obtaining a measure of hypnotic responsivity include the following. If someone is highly hypnotizable, the absence of an induction ceremony does not mean that spontaneous trances have not taken place (e.g., Frankel, 1975), for example, during interrogation, interviews, or through the use of imagery techniques that elicit hypnotic responses, even though a clinician did not use the word "hypnosis." In fact, under motivated or pressured conditions, highly hypnotizable persons may be more prone to enter a hypnotic state (Spiegel, 1974, 1980). Conversely, just because an induction ceremony was conducted, does not mean that the person was hypnotized. Finally, some persons believe there may be a need to work more carefully with highly hypnotizable persons due to their potential to accept ideas uncritically and to confabulate (Orne, 1979). Because high hypnotizable persons appear to be the population most likely to manifest dissociative phenomena, therapists also may need to work extra cautiously with these patients. Standardized procedures with norms and known psychometric properties will become especially important in the forensic setting because they comply with Daubert ruling criteria for something testable, repeatable, and falsifiable (*Daubert v. Merrell Dow Pharmaceuticals, Inc.*, 125 L.Ed.2d 469, 1993).

Awareness of the level of hypnotic responsivity of a patient also alerts the clinician to those individuals who may have greater potential vulnerability for pseudomemory production in or out of hypnosis. In situations involving allegations that therapists have encouraged the production of false memories, documentation that the patient scores lower in hypnotizability, and in interrogative suggestibility (Gudjonsson, 1984, 1992), may provide some supportive corroboration that the patient was not someone who would be anticipated to have a high likelihood for developing pseudomemories. In someone with lower suggestibility, there is a much lower likelihood that the suggestions of a therapist were accepted. Thus, in People v. Caro (1988) a low hypnotizability score was found to be evidence that even though a hypnotic induction ceremony had been performed, the witness was not hypnotized.

It is very important, however, that the capacity for accepting hypnotic or other suggestions should not be considered to be directly correlated with the likelihood that a particular memory is true or false. In other words, the fact that a person scores high on hypnotic or interrogative suggestibility scales does not prove that their memories are false. At the opposite end of the continuum, people with low suggestibility should likewise not be assumed to have only real memories. No matter what the suseptibility level, there is no substitute for independent corroboration. Performance on suggestibility scales is most useful in assessing the possibility of a suggestion having been accepted. It has nothing to do with whether an alleged memory is actually true or false. It is simply useful in helping us search for the source of the memory.

6. Documentation and Record Keeping

The more serious or unusual the memories and allegations of a patient, the more thorough the treatment notes should be. Chart notes should document discussions of hypnosis and memory, issues of accuracy of memory, informed consent, and the maintenance of a stance of neutrality and the avoidance of offering definite opinions in the absence of corroborating evidence. Chart notes should also document efforts to encourage critical evaluation of hypnotically elicited material, and discouragement of confrontation with alleged perpetrators, and the potential negative ramifications of such confrontation. In the event that legal issues arise, it is recommended that the therapist consult legal counsel.

7. Inquiry During Hypnosis

Patients should be instructed that questions will be asked that should not be interpreted as suggestions, but as an inquiries for information. They may only say what they have said before, it may be different, or it may be new, or some combination of the above. If they do not have an answer, this is an acceptable response. The therapist must be careful to remain nonleading (Mutter, 1984).

Following initial suggestions for age regression, clinicians should allow the patient to engage in relatively free recall, with minimal questioning concerning the content of the memory until it has been thoroughly elaborated by the patient. Questions about specific content and details should only follow the completion of a free narrative report by the patient. During the initial recall, therapists may wish to ask specific but nonleading questions that inquire about the feelings the subject is experiencing. Likewise, the therapist may sometimes simply repeat patient phrases verbatim to acknowledge hearing the statement of the patient, or may offer comments that encourage the patient to continue (e.g., "Um-hmm," "Yes," "Go on," "What are you aware of?" "Are you aware of anything else?" "Does anything else occur?") Prior to questioning about content or the use of working through techniques, patients may also be asked to return to the beginning of the event and to quietly review it for several minutes (Mutter, 1990). Be aware that information retrieved may not be veridical, but simply what the patient believes to be true.

The confidence displayed by subjects in material retrieved under hypnosis can influence the therapist's belief in the accuracy of the information. There is thus a reciprocal influence process, and it seems imperative that therapists must be warned that confidence on the part of the patient or affective intensity does not mean that recalled material is accurate, and should not lead to the acceptance of the information reported as veridical in nature. Events that are imagined in hypnosis may stir emotions and have a quality of reality and genuineness, especially if they meet the preconceptions or satisfy the emotional needs of the patient, as well as if they are reinforced by the therapist. Likewise, when something is remembered with partial accuracy but in a somewhat fuzzy manner that may not be entirely comprehensible, it is possible that subjects may reconstruct or add to this material in ways of which they are not aware in an effort to make it meaningful, understandable, complete or consistent.

The hypnotic technique of ideomotor signaling, while not a truth serum nor a direct line to the unconscious, may be useful in both clinical and investigative hypnosis in providing another source of information to be balanced with material already in conscious awareness. Ideomotor signals may also be used in lieu of verbal responses. There is some disagreement in the hypnosis community as to the value of the ideomotor signaling technique. Although there are numerous case reports, and three experimental studies of chemically dissociated memory (two reported by Bennett, 1988, and Rath, 1982), that have provided support for the plausible value of ideomotor signaling, further studies with ecological validity (conducted with personally meaningful and emotional or traumatic memories) should be conducted on this, as well as other hypnotic exploration techniques. However, leading or suggestive questions may be asked improperly with this or any other hypnotic technique, just as they may be in nonhypnotic interviews. Suggestive questions may sometimes be part of promoting symptomatic change. But in any investigative or forensic context, or for memory retrieval in any form, clinicians must be cautious not to frame questions in a leading manner, whether they are requesting verbal or nonverbal responses. In this regard, in using ideomotor signals, we believe it is less leading when inquiring concerning memory to use four signals, as originally advocated by Cheek and LeCron (1968), for "yes," "no," "I don't want to say," and for "I don't know."

However, irrespective of what hypnotic method is used, or whether a "memory" has been spontaneously recalled by a patient, what is most important to realize is that we have no validated litmus test to distinguish genuine from false or partially accurate memories. Therefore, the bottom line is that in the absence of some kind of corroborative evidence, therapists should not convey acceptance of the accuracy of material uncovered with any hypnotic technique. Because persons in hypnosis may not critically evaluate data elicited in hypnosis, it is important to assist them to do so in psychotherapy interviews following hypnotic uncovering. Treatment of traumatic memories involves more than simply bypassing traumatic amnesia. Information elicited must be critically examined outside hypnosis and integrated in an ego-syntonic way.

8. Use of Dissociative Regression Techniques

There are hypnotic procedures referred to as dissociative regression techniques. Such methods (some of which are reviewed in Hammond, 1990) are used to assist patients in recalling and working through traumatic material of an intense emotional nature, but in a manner that titrates affect and avoids overwhelming the patient. Thus, the goal of such techniques is therapeutic and helpful. These methods include techniques such as viewing a traumatic event from a distance or on a screen, the fractionated abreaction (wherein the full event is processed gradually in a start-stop-start-stop manner) (Kluft, 1990), dissociating affect and content, and giving suggestions for time distortion to speed up the recall of a memory and minimize patient suffering. Ideomotor signals are likewise sometimes used to inquire about the emotions involved in an event, prior to remembering it, to ease a patient closer to potentially intense material. The other method uses ideomotor signals in a careful, non-leading manner to identify potential content associated with a memory prior to age regression. For example, someone may be asked, "Was there anyone else present with you at the time of this event? Was there more than one other person? Was it a male? Was it a female? Was it someone you knew? Was it a member of your immediate or extended family?"

It is not known definitively what degree of distortion may be introduced by the use of dissociative regression techniques, but we believe that such methods may have some potential to alter a memory to at least some degree. We must await research to determine whether distortion is encouraged by such methods in a clinical population with traumatic memories. But, when a screen or television technique is used, for example, patients are being asked to use their imagination and see an event differently. This has the inherent risk or potential of altering a memory in ways currently unspecified by research.

While awaiting such clinically relevant research, we recommend that therapists and patients collaboratively make decisions about the use of these methods, balancing the patient's emotional well being with the need for historical accuracy. In some cases (e.g., where a court case is not pending or anticipated, an alleged perpetrator is already in prison or deceased, or the patient already remembers the traumatic event that remains to be worked through), dissociative regression techniques may be very appropriate and therapeutic. But, when screen techniques are used, it should not be implied that the mind remembers everything as if recorded on a videotape, and should not, therefore, suggest that the person can "zoom in" and will be able to see or hear anything that occurred. Such a method creates demands on the patient and provides permission to imaginatively fantasize and confabulate information that may have never been recorded in memory (e.g., because the person was too far away to see or hear anything).

9. Supportiveness to Patients

Perceived rejection by a therapist has been found to be associated with destructive effects (Lieberman, Yalom & Miles, 1973). As helping professionals, we do not want to harm victims of alleged abuse by being perceived as rejecting and disbelieving their productions, particularly when at least the broad outlines of what they recall (with or without hypnosis) might be genuine. There is abundant evidence that abuse is widespread. At the same time, however, no one would wish to harm innocent people through encouraging impulsive or premature accusation where there is an absence of confirming evidence.

But, a stance of silence or uninvolved impartiality may be perceived as rejection by patients. Thus, in the interests of being therapeutic, we need to demonstrate a balance between supportiveness and empathic understanding, while at the same time assisting the patient in a nonhypnotized state to critically evaluate the material elicited with hypnosis. We must simultaneously convey openness and support, while still assuming a stance that memory is frequently imperfect and that rarely will all the details of any recollection be fully accurate. Since we were not actually present ourselves in the original situation being recalled, we cannot guarantee to patients that what was remembered is accurate. We should believe in our patients and express faith in them, while remembering that having faith in a patient is not synonymous with always believing everything a patient believes or produces. Both therapist and patient should regard material elicited under hypnosis as simply one more source of information that cannot be relied on as superior to or more accurate than material already in conscious awareness. It is simply further information to be weighed along with data and feelings already consciously available to the patient, while tolerating ambiguity and avoiding or even challenging premature closure (Wells & Leippe, 1981). Therapists should maintain an openness to potential alternative explanations for the production of a "memory," including family or personal dynamics, or possible secondary gains (e.g., as a face saving excuse, for revenge). Likewise, when there are blocks to memory that have the appearance of amnesia, inquiry should be made concerning organic factors (e.g., alcohol or drug use, illness, blows to the head) that may potentially account for substantial lapses in memory. It is also incumbent upon therapists to realize that even when material recalled in therapy cannot be independently confirmed, it may nonetheless be influential.

In an effort to control for possible contamination, it is suggested that group therapies of a kind allowing discussion of past history or abuse (but not professionally conducted groups that are highly structured and focused on the acquisition of coping skills), may be most appropriate later in the treatment of victims of abuse.

10. Inappropriate Confrontation & Issues of Litigation

It is inappropriate and goes beyond proper therapeutic roles and boundaries to encourage patients to institute litigation. Therapists should caution patients against impulsive actions of any kind based on information uncovered in hypnosis, encouraging them to thoughtfully and critically evaluate this material for a substantial period of time, as well as potential negative consequences of confrontation or disclosure of this information. These cautions and actions should be documented in the patient's chart. We consider it to be improper to encourage patients to confront alleged perpetrators based solely on information retrieved under hypnosis. Furthermore, suggesting a confrontation or inviting family members into one's office to discuss such matters essentially gives family members the status of patients, increasing the duty owed and one's potential legal liability. As a member of the False Memory Syndrome Foundation advisory board (Frankel, 1994) wrote: "What is essential to the clinical work is that the product of the inquiry remains in the treatment context; it is not essential that veridicality be established. When the content is taken out of the clinical office into the home of ageing parents 20-30 years after an alleged trauma, or into the courts, the situation becomes complicated and is in fact beyond the competence of many clinicians." In working with children, therapists may be bound by law to report allegations of child abuse, but there is no increased credibility of a child's statement over that of an adult, and it should be conveyed to authorities that the account was based on hypnotically elicited recall and that the allegation by the child may not be accurate.

If a patient does decide independently, outside of the context of therapy, to confront an alleged abuser, it is critically important for the therapist to clarify in writing that the confrontation was done against the advice of the therapist and does not create any type of therapeutic relationship between the therapist and alleged abuser. This may take the form of a written and signed statement by the patient which acknowledges that the therapist has advised that such a confrontation may be emotionally distressing to both the alleged abuser and the patient.

11. Cautions

Finally, we believe that there may be certain situations that should perhaps raise a "red flag" in a therapist's mind concerning the possible validity of a recovered memory, encouraging extra circumspection. The following items are based primarily on clinical intuition rather than established research, and should be regarded strictly as situations where we encourage cautiousness on the part of therapists, and not as circumstances where it is impossible that a recalled memory has validity.

A. A patient with a history of switching therapists or doctor shopping. It may be wise to have such patients provide a detailed history of prior therapy in their own handwriting and to provide a release of information for all prior therapists. A patient unwilling to do this may not want unfavorable information in prior treatment records to be available.

B. When the possibility of litigation is raised, especially early in therapy or when an attorney has been consulted prior to the onset of therapy. Similarly, when the patient demonstrates an overfamiliarity with psychological terminology and litigation concepts, it implies substantial prior experience that should be explored by the therapist.

C. In the treatment of highly manipulative patients with characterological issues.

D. Caution should be exercised in uncritically accepting memories in a patient coming for treatment to "confirm" if he/she were abused in the past. The therapist cannot make that determination without independent factual corroboration. The therapist cannot act as a judge or jury.

E. Caution should be observed when a previous therapist has suggested that abuse may have occurred.

F. When uncovered memories are from before the age of 3.

G. In persons remembering amnestic memories from adolescence or adulthood, or who claim to have a lack of memories for significant blocks of time after the middle of childhood, but who do not demonstrate evidence of a dissociative disorder on objective evaluation (e.g., with the Dissociative Experiences Scale, the SCID-D, and the HIP) (Bernstein & Putnam, 1986; Frischholz, Lipman, Braun, & Sachs, 1992; Steinberg, 1994; Steinberg, Cicchetti, Buchanan, Hall, & Rounsaville, 1993).

H. In instances where the past relationship with the alleged perpetrator was an entirely positive one, not associated with ambivalent feelings, aloofness or conflicts.

I. When patients have previously seen unlicensed therapists or lay hypnotists. Likewise, extra caution is indicated when a previous therapist has used non-traditional forms of therapy, such as (but not limited to) crystals, energy balancing, muscle testing, reading auras, past life therapy, or expelling entities from the patient. In such circumstances, we believe the potential for patients to be inappropriately influenced in their expectations and to misunderstand and misinterpret such techniques is much higher.

J. When patients have participated in lay support or self-help groups which are unsupervised by licensed professionals, and where a topic of discussion is often trauma, sexual abuse, or incest. Likewise, extra caution is indicated when the patient's memories are subject to contamination because the patient has participated in seminars on abuse, read literature on abuse, or viewed television or video presentations on abuse.

K. When the therapist has a personal history similar to the patient, potentially leading to the increased possibility of unconscious bias, misinterpretation, and countertransference.

On the other hand, one may speculate that there may likewise be situations where therapists may tentatively consider the recovered memories of patients as possibly having more validity, such as when memories return outside of a therapeutic interview or more spontaneously, when someone else reported abuse by the same perpetrator, when the patients journal or diaries described the forgotten abuse, and when the patient is able to pinpoint specific "triggers" that they believe elicited the recall of a memory (and the memory is very similar to the situation or cues that evoked it) outside of hypnosis. One might also be tempted to speculate that a recovered memory might have more validity when the patient recalling abuse has always had memories of other abuse within the family or by the alleged perpetrator. However, the research on pseudomemories might suggest that perhaps this latter kind of person, because he or she would perceive the event as having a relatively high base rate of occurrence, may be even more vulnerable to pseudomemory creation. The reality is that speculations such as these must still be identified as nothing more than conjecture and unvalidated hypotheses, because we do not yet have a way to reliably determine the validity of memories.

There is much we still do not know about memory and about memory and hypnosis. Therapists must be aware of the memory research and recommendations for the conduct of forensic hypnosis, and that memory is somewhat malleable and can be influenced either through conscious interrogation, suggestion and interviewing techniques, or through suggestive hypnotic techniques. There is a time for suggestion in hypnosis, but that time is not during the initial elicitation and uncovering of memories.

Summary of the A.S.C.H. Recommendations for Clinicians Working With Hypnosis and Memory With Potential Victims of Abuse

1. Prior to hypnosis, evaluate the patient and explore his/her expectations about hypnosis. When there are beliefs that abuse may have occurred, evaluate potential sources of contamination (e.g., referral sources, reading, groups, seminars, T.V., persons with similar experiences).

2. Age regression and uncovering techniques in hypnosis should only be used by licensed health and mental health professionals, within their areas of expertise. Prior to using hypnotic uncovering methods, health professionals should have received systematic training in hypnosis, meeting at least the minimum standards set forth in the A.S.C.H. Standards of Training in Clinical Hypnosis (Hammond & Elkins, 1994), be familiar with the literature on hypnosis and memory, have competency in avoiding leading questions in and out of hypnosis, and have psychotherapeutic training in working with victims of abuse or trauma.

3. Informed consent should be obtained prior to induction of hypnosis, except in unusual (e.g., medical emergency) situations, informing patients of potential limitation of rights to testify if hypnosis is performed, and discussing that memory is imperfect. Hypnotic uncovering is dangerous if not contraindicated in patients with fragile ego-strength, extreme emotional lability, tenuous control, thought disorder, and with some medically impaired patients.

4. To minimize errors of creating false confidence, neutral expectations should be created both prior to hypnosis, and during hypnotic induction and age regression. This neutrality should structure patient expectations to the effect that further information may or may not be forthcoming, and may or may not be accurate. It should not be suggested that "everything has been recorded in your mind, nothing has been forgotten, and it will now be freely accessible and you can and will clearly remember everything." Therapists who have themselves been victims of abuse should exercise particular caution to ensure that their own abuse issues have been adequately resolved.

5. It is recommended in working with potential victims of abuse that therapists evaluate hypnotic responsivity, at least informally. It may be advisable to consider obtaining a formal measure of hypnotic responsivity to document the level of hypnotizability and determine the likelihood that the person was actually hypnotized. Performance on suggestibility scales is useful in assessing the possibility that a suggestion may have been accepted, but it has nothing to do with whether an alleged memory is actually true or false. Because high hypnotizable persons appear to be the population most likely to manifest dissociative phenomena, therapists should work extra cautiously with these patients.

6. The more serious or unusual the memories and allegations of a patient, the more thorough the treatment notes should be. Chart notes should document discussions of hypnosis and memory, issues of accuracy of memory, informed consent, and the maintenance of a stance of neutrality and the avoidance of offering definite opinions in the absence of corroborating evidence. In the event that legal issues arise, it is recommended that therapists consult legal counsel.

7. Patients should be instructed to not interpret questions as suggestions, but as an inquiries, and that if they do not have an answer, this is an acceptable response. Following age regression, allow the patient to engage in relatively free recall until the memory has been thoroughly elaborated, with minimal nonleading questioning concerning the content of the memory, simple repetition of patient phrases verbatim, or comments that simply encourage the patient to continue. Realize that confidence or affective intensity does not mean that recalled material is accurate, and that we have no validated test to distinguish genuine from false or partially accurate memories. In the absence of some kind of corroborative evidence, therapists should not convey acceptance of the accuracy of uncovered material. Because persons in hypnosis may not critically evaluate elicited material, assist them to do so in subsequent psychotherapy interviews.

8. Dissociative age regression techniques may assist patients in recalling and working through intense traumatic material, but it is not known what degree of distortion may be introduced by such techniques. They may have some potential to alter a memory and, therefore, decisions about the use of these methods should balance the emotional well being of the patient with the need for historical accuracy.

9. We do not want to harm victims of alleged abuse by having them perceive us as rejecting because we disbelieve their productions. At the same time, however, no one wishes to harm innocent people through encouraging impulsive or premature accusation in the absence of confirming evidence. Demonstrate a balance between supportiveness and empathy, while at the same time assisting patients in a nonhypnotized state to critically evaluate material elicited. Both therapist and patient should regard material elicited under hypnosis as simply one more source of information that cannot be relied on as superior to or more accurate than material already in conscious awareness. We can believe in patients without necessarily believing everything they produce.

10. It is inappropriate to encourage patients to institute litigation or to confront alleged perpetrators based solely on information retrieved under hypnosis.

SECTION 4

RECOMMENDATIONS FOR THE CONDUCT OF FORENSIC HYPNOSIS

Recommendations for clinical and forensic interviews are not mutually exclusive. The committee has reviewed literature and finds that the subsequent recommendations are applicable for the forensic interview. At present there are two different forensic models which have been in operational use. The first is the "federal" model, originally drafted for the FBI (Ault, 1979, 1980; Garver, 1987), but now used by many federal agencies. The second model was originally drafted by Martin T. Orne (Orne, 1979) and is known either as the Orne guidelines or the *Hurd* guidelines based upon the New Jersey Supreme Court adoption in 1981 (*State v. Hurd,* 1981). In the recommendations that follow, the committee will make appropriate references to both the federal and state models. The committee has added additional recommendations deemed to be important in the investigative/legal process for the protection of the witness/defendant. The professional conducting forensic hypnosis under these guidelines should also be familiar with the Recommendations for Clinicians Working with Hypnosis and Memory.

1. Responsibility and Qualifications

The investigative hypnosis process should be the responsibility of the mental health professional (as defined or authorized by existing statutes or judicial rulings) with knowledge of the literature on memory and hypnosis, and on memory. The professional should also have demonstrated competence and training in hypnosis (Hammond & Elkins, 1994), forensic applications of hypnosis, and nonsuggestive interviewing/interrogation.

It is the responsibility of the licensed mental health professional to reject the use of hypnosis in any case in which:

a. The witness was not in a position to realistically perceive the events in question.
b. The use of hypnosis appears to pose a risk of harm to the mental, emotional or physical health status of the person.
c. The witness is not competent to give informed consent.
d. The witness does not give written informed consent.

The above is consistent with state model guidelines.

2. Decision to Use Forensic Hypnosis & Informed Consent

Because the use of hypnosis may have further ramifications, the decision to utilize a hypnotic interview should be undertaken only after other traditional law enforcement procedures have been employed (Hibler, 1984). The mental health professional should also inquire of the police, prosecutor, or defense counsel as to the latest rulings concerning forensic hypnosis in that jurisdiction.

It is important that the investigator working as a hypnotic coordinator with the hypnotherapist has been cautious to assure that the case has no investigative failures, as might be seen in wrongly exposing the hypnotic interviewee to a suspect at an earlier time, thus violating rules of conduct for eyewitness identification and contaminating the witness for hypnotic purposes.

The investigators or attorney should provide the mental health professional with a brief written summary of the case and objectives for the forensic use of hypnosis. The written information should not provide details that would allow the mental health professional to unduly lead the subject, but it should contain a sufficient amount of information to help determine the appropriateness of using hypnosis in the individual case.

The mental health professional will obtain written informed consent from the witness or his/her guardian or legal representative, where applicable. A copy of the recommended form for informed consent in a forensic setting is reproduced in Appendix B. The witness should be informed that he/she may terminate the hypnotic interview at any time if he/she should so desire. The informed consent should include a statement holding the mental health professional harmless if the hypnotically obtained information is later deemed to be inadmissible. This guideline is consistent with both the federal and the state model.

3. Role & Involvement of Other Persons in Forensic Interviews

The federal and state guidelines are not in agreement on the issue of who may be present in the room while the interview is being conducted.

A. *The Federal Model.* The number of people present in the room during the interview should be kept to a minimum, but may include the prosecuting and/or defense attorneys, the case agent, a police artist, a chaperon when appropriate, or a close friend or family member at the request of the interviewee. While conducting the interview, the consultation team should be careful not to prompt the witness verbally or nonverbally with any new components to the description of his/her experience and should be especially careful not to alter the perceptual reality of the incident in any way.

When using a team approach, the law enforcement officer must have received specific training to assist in hypnotic interviews. The mental health professional is in complete charge of the process to protect the mental well being of the interviewee. Following hypnotic induction and regression, the investigator is in charge of the questioning. In certain circumstances, the mental health professional may also make inquiry. However, care must be taken, regardless of who is conducting the interview, to avoid undue suggestion or contamination. In the event that the questioning may produce undue stress, which may compromise the emotional health or legal rights of the interviewee, the mental health professional can terminate the interview and bring the interviewee out of hypnosis.

B. *The State Model.* The state model differs wherein only the interviewee and the mental health professional are in the room exclusively. A police artist may be called in at a later time.

Experience has demonstrated that while the purpose of this restriction, to avoid an additional source of undue suggestion, is legitimate, it may be overweighed by the more important consideration of protecting the witness/defendant's mental well being and legal rights. Therefore, in appropriate cases (e.g., where female rape victims will be hypnotized by a male hypnotist), with consent of the prosecuting attorney, it may be determined that the witness/defendant's primary therapist, prosecuting or defense attorney, case agent, police artist, chaperon when appropriate, or a close friend or family member might be allowed to be present in the room. Their mere presence in the room, without the exertion of any influence or suggestion, may be of great comfort and concern to the witness/defendant and may, therefore, facilitate better hypnotic recall. But, if such individuals are present in the room, they must be told not to speak and to avoid nonverbal communications. Any communication should be in written form to the interviewer, and these notes must be preserved in the file.

C. *Hypnosis with Defendants.* It is impermissible under both the federal and state guidelines for police to hypnotically interview suspects or defendants. In the event where a defense attorney is seeking additional information from his/her client, an independent mental health professional may be employed to interview and hypnotize a defendant. The mental health professional must follow these recommended guidelines (Mutter, 1990). The defense attorney may be present or in a monitoring room and may write questions in the latter phases of the hypnotic interview.

4. Video & Audio Taping

In the federal and state models making a videotape recording of the interview is mandatory. (A checklist of information to consider when preparing for the interview appears in Appendix C.) Prior to the interview, the equipment should be thoroughly double checked to ensure that the equipment is in good working order, and that there are sufficient video and audiotapes available. It is recommended that several different microphones be available. The video and audiotaping should begin at the outset of the interview and be made continuously, with a time period generator documenting this continuous recording, and all persons present in the room should be on camera.

5. Conduct of the Forensic Interview Prior to Hypnosis

After obtaining written informed consent, rapport should be established with the patient. A psychiatric/psychological evaluation (such as a mental status examination, medical history, prior psychiatric history, or other pertinent data) should be obtained from the interviewee prior to hypnosis, and this should also be videotaped. The witness/defendant should also be asked if he/she has any questions before the hypnotic interview begins.

Next, a free narrative recall should be obtained to preserve the prehypnotic recollections of the witness. For example, "Tell me what you remember." Specific questions for detailed information should be avoided at this time. At the conclusion of the free narrative, the witness may be asked to pause for a moment, and to then see if there is any additional information remembered. At this point, more specific, but non-leading questions may be asked. The witness may be asked to provide a pictorial diagram of the event or scene of the event. A description at this time may be given to a police artist to obtain a sketch of any person or object. The witness may be asked to describe any previous statements he or she has given to police or other individuals. The witness may be asked to recall what he or she has been told by others, or what they may have read or seen in the news media, where applicable. Memorializing prehypnotic recall on videotape is vitally important because research (Whitehouse, Orne, Orne & Dinges, 1991) suggests that without this, witnesses may not always be able to reliably distinguish between memories retrieved prior to hypnosis and those that occurred during hypnosis.

If at this point, the use of hypnosis is indicated, information should be obtained concerning any physical limitations, such as visual or hearing impairments. The witness may then be educated about the nature of hypnosis, and questions may be answered about hypnosis. Witness expectations about the nature of hypnosis and the influence of hypnosis on memory should be elicited, and misconceptions clarified. This education should include acknowledgement that memory is imperfect in or out of hypnosis and all demand characteristics regarding memory retrieval should be avoided. It is important that the witness understand that memory does not act as a tape recorder, and that new information may or may not be remembered with hypnosis, and may or may not be accurate. Thus, neutral prehypnotic expectations are structured.

6. Use of Objective Tests of Hypnotic Responsivity

From 1923 to 1993, the law generally followed the *Frye* rule on admissibility of expert opinion testimony (*Frye*, 1923). According to the *Frye* rule, when an expert bases an opinion upon a scientific technique, instrumentality, modality or procedure, "the thing from which the deduction is made must be sufficiently established to have gained general acceptance in the particular [scientific] field in which it belongs" (*Frye*, 1923). The *Frye* test generally tended to exclude testimony that was *relevant*, but not *reliable*. [When the Supreme Court talks about "reliability," it generally means what scientists would call validity.]

In June 1993, the United States Supreme Court decided *Daubert v. Merrell Dow Pharmaceuticals, Inc.*, 125 L.Ed.2d 469 (1993). *Daubert* held that the landmark *Frye* test for the admissibility of expert opinion testimony would no longer govern in federal courts. In its place is a new test, found in Federal Rules of Evidence, Rule 702, which states: "If scientific, technical, or other specialized knowledge will assist the trier of fact to understand the evidence or to determine a fact in issue, a witness qualified as an expert by knowledge, skill, experience, training, or education, may testify thereto in the form of an opinion or otherwise."

This new test follows what the Court considered the "baseline" for the admissibility of all evidence, which it found in Rule 402's statement that "all relevant evidence is admissible...." Thus, the new test under the Federal Rules of Evidence places emphasis on *relevance*, rather than on reliability. It appears likely that the following two consequences will result from *Daubert:*

First, many, if not most, states will replace the *Frye* rule with the more lenient "relevance" test. Second, when the issues of admissibility of hypnotically refreshed recollection are reviewed in state and federal courts, evidence that would have been ruled inadmissible under the *Frye* rule will now be permitted under the more liberal "relevance" test.

It is likely that the majority of states presently following the *per se* exclusion rule regarding hypnotically refreshed testimony will be urged by law enforcement, clinicians, and others to repeal these restrictive anti-hypnosis holdings in favor of the adoption of a rule favoring admissibility (Scheflin, 1994a, 1994b).

Though the new test adopted in *Daubert* places emphasis on "relevance," it does not reject "reliability." In addressing this last point, the Supreme Court noted that opinion testimony must count on "scientific knowledge." In order to do so, the "proposed testimony must be supported by appropriate validation--i.e., 'good grounds,' based on what is known. In short, the requirement that an expert's testimony pertain to 'scientific knowledge' establishes a standard of evidentiary reliability."

In a footnote, the Court further added that "in a case involving scientific evidence, evidentiary reliability will be based upon scientific validity." A majority of the Court used terms like "validity," "falsifiability," and "testability" when discussing the issue of reliability. Trial judges will acknowledge these terms when assessing the reliability of expert opinion testimony.

Even before the *Daubert* ruling, some courts have based their decisions on the weight given to such tests (*People v. Caro,* 1988; *People v. Johnson,* 1989). It seems reasonable to conclude that the *Daubert* case encourages the use of objective tests, or a preliminary hypnotic evaluation eliciting phenomena of established difficulty level, in forensic hypnosis interviews.

Some members of this committee, as well as others in the fields of psychology and psychiatry, have done clinical and experimental research which produced valid and reliable instruments to measure hypnotic capacity and responsivity. These members feel strongly that the state of the art in clinical measurement has reached a point where it should become mandatory, even without *Daubert,* to use standardized instruments (e.g., the Hypnotic Induction Profile, the Stanford Scales) in addition to informal assessments which are not subject to test-retest or interrater reliability and validity criteria. While such informal tests may have some clinical usefulness, these committee members believe that by themselves they fall short of *Daubert's* quest to establish relevance *and* reliability based on scientific criteria of testability, verification, and falsifiability.

Many forensic hypnosis experts have raised objections to objective testing. These experts point out that the objective tests need better validation on traumatized populations. Although some studies of hypnotic responsivity in post-traumatic stress disorder populations exist (Spiegel, Hunt, & Dondershine, 1988; Stutman & Bliss, 1985), it is important that more data be developed concerning these tests among victims of a wider range of traumatic stressors.

Other committee members believe that it is unnecessary to utilize standardized measures in forensic cases, and that informal evaluation of responsivity is sufficient. Therefore, given the difference of opinion in this area, the committee concludes that it may thus be advisable for experts in forensic hypnosis to receive training in, and to consider utilizing, standardized hypnotizability measurements, scales and tests, but there is a division among the committee that this should be required at this time. All of the committee is in agreement, however, that such testing of hypnotic responsivity, or the use of a preliminary trance evaluation (that elicits hypnotic phenomena of known difficulty level) to ascertain hypnotic responsivity, does not constitute a trance for legal purposes, nor should it be regarded as a contaminant because it is content-free with regard to exploration of potential memories relevant to the investigation.

7. The Existence of Spontaneous Trance Without Formal Hypnosis

The committee acknowledges that highly hypnotizable individuals are believed to enter trance states spontaneously, without a formal induction (Beahrs, 1988). Courts have not addressed this phenomenon yet, but the literature suggests that this may occur during nonhypnotic interrogation. This underscores the potential importance of hypnotizability assessment by a trained mental health professional who may assist in determining the probability that trance states may have occurred spontaneously during previous nonhypnotic interrogations. The mental health professional may, therefore, be in a position to assess the legal implications.

8. The Hypnosis Interview

Following any standardized hypnotizability testing or informal trance evaluation that may be conducted, a hypnotic induction for the hypnotic interview is conducted and hypnotic phenomena may be elicited to further document responsivity or depth. Age or time regression is then performed, initially allowing free recall, following the format described in clinical guideline 7. The mental health professional assumes responsibility for the management of the interviewee's affective reactions, modulating these as necessary for the well being of the witness/defendant. However, dissociative regression techniques must be used cautiously in a forensic interview to avoid undue suggestion.

Following free recall, the interviewee may be questioned further, using either verbal recall (hypermnesia and/or revivification) and/or ideomotor signaling. Since information in investigative hypnosis interviews must always be independently corroborated, following free recall, there may be selected cases where it is not unreasonable to "push the limits" and give suggestions that instill confidence that more information will be remembered, or also use screen techniques. An illustration of where this might be appropriate would be in a kidnapping case where further investigative leads are needed, and where time is of the essence. However, when working with defendants, the interviewer must always bear in mind that there may be increased motivation for the interviewee to produce self-serving information (intentionally or unintentionally), or to feign hypnosis.

In jurisdictions where a case agent, investigator, or attorney/prosecutor may legally be involved in the interview process, they should be present throughout the interview. Such individuals may pass on notes to the mental health professional or person conducting the interview during the inquiry phase of the interview. The purpose of such communication is to specify factors which are of importance to the case, but which may not have been otherwise developed in the inquiry. The interviewer needs to be careful in phrasing questions prompted by such notes, so as not to suggest conclusions reached by investigators. Further, such notes should be retained in the case file.

Breaks may be needed to change the tape, use the lavatory, or possibly allow for meals. Hypnosis should be terminated before breaks, and on tape a precautionary statement made that the case is not to be discussed on break. In a team approach, the mental health professional is responsible for terminating or re-initiating hypnosis as needed. After realerting, the mental health professional should arrange for any clinical follow-up that may be needed to address mental health needs of the witness. The forensic consultant should not be the person to provide any therapeutic follow-up. In cases where the witness is in therapy, permission may be obtained to provide therapeutic input to the therapist.

If new descriptions were obtained in hypnosis, have the interviewee report them again following the termination of hypnosis. A posthypnotic suggestion by the mental health professional may also be given to assist in providing recall of the descriptions out of hypnosis. Following re-alerting at the end of the interview, the mental health professional should check for any sequelae of hypnosis, and obtain input about the subjective experience of the interviewee that may provide further data. After the witness/defendant is realerted, before stopping the videotaping, the interviewee should be asked "How do you feel?" Do not stop the taping until the witness/defendant indicates that she/he is okay. The mental health professional should also dictate a short statement at the conclusion of the interview to detail the procedure utilized and his/her observations during the session (e.g., depth of trance, phenomena elicited, hypnotizability score), and his/her opinion regarding the validity of the hypnotic state. This note should be maintained with the case file and a copy kept by the mental health professional.

9. Self-Incriminating Statements

During forensic hypnosis, if the interviewee incriminates him/herself, the mental health consultant should terminate hypnosis, have the interviewee acknowledge verbally that he/she is out of trance, and the law enforcement investigator or attorney will advise the interviewee of his/her rights. In the state model, a defendant may make a self-incriminating statement. When working with defendants, the function of the interviewer is to seek additional data that may explain the behavior involved in a criminal act.

10. Hypnosis is Not More Distorting Than Other Retrieval Methods

Experimental research evidence demonstrates that any form of memory retrieval, when used improperly, may contaminate memory. Many courts have had the mistaken idea that simply because hypnosis was used, memory must, therefore, have been contaminated. In fact, however, when hypnosis is used properly, there is no evidence to suggest that it is any more likely to contaminate memory than any other properly used memory retrieval technique. Nonhypnotic variables have been shown to produce significant memory contaminations.

Similar memory contaminations have been found when using these nonhypnotic variables (e.g., leading questions) in conjunction with hypnosis. Thus, hypnosis, when used properly, does not appear to make a unique contribution to the memory contamination process. In the conduct of the forensic interview, before, during, and following hypnosis, the forensic hypnosis team should be sensitive to avoid leading questions, and verbal or nonverbal suggestions that may distort or alter recall of the incident being investigated.

11. Posthypnotic Evaluation

The hypnotic interview should be discussed with investigating officers or attorneys following the session. Discussion should note the potential limitations of additional material that was obtained, and that all information must be independently corroborated for it to have credibility. Afterwards, a written report should be provided or dictated, including details about the hypnotic techniques used, observations during the session (e.g., depth of trance, phenomena elicited, hypnotizability score), and opinions concerning the validity of the hypnotic state. Any departures from these recommended procedures, and the reasons such deviations occurred, should also be noted. A case officer or attorney may wish to note any new information that was elicited.

APPENDIX A

SAMPLE INFORMED CONSENT DOCUMENT

The following informed consent documents are offered as a sample for clinicians to consider. The sample informed consent forms should not be construed as the most appropriate form in all instances and it may be necessary to approach differing circumstances or legal jurisdictions with a different form than outlined here. Thus, therapists may wish to consult legal counsel regarding the rulings of legal authorities in their jurisdiction.

HYPNOSIS: LEGAL CONSEQUENCES

INFORMED CONSENT

The Nature of Hypnosis. Memory is imperfect, whether or not hypnosis is used. Memory is not like a tape recorder, and rarely will all the details of any recollection be fully accurate. People have been shown to be capable of filling in gaps in memory, of distorting information, and of being influenced in what is "remembered" by leading questions or suggestions. For example, our memories may sometimes be influenced through reading, movies, TV, or conversations. Thus, research has shown that there is no guarantee that information remembered through hypnosis (or through ordinary recall) is factually accurate. On the other hand, information that is so remembered through hypnosis may in fact be accurate. But, the only way one may know definitively whether something recalled under hypnosis is accurate is to obtain independent corroboration. Thus, if you should remember something under hypnosis, regard this information as simply one more source of data that cannot be relied on as more accurate or necessarily superior to material already in conscious awareness. Such further data would simply be information to be weighed and evaluated in therapy along with what you already consciously know.

Potential Legal Issue. In many jurisdictions, courts have held that a person who has been hypnotized cannot testify in court about anything remembered during or after the hypnosis. Consequently, if I consent to hypnosis, there is a possibility that anything I remember once the hypnosis begins will not be admissible in a court of law. The only way to fully protect my potential right to testify is to forego the use of hypnosis.

Release from Liability. I understand that, because of the rulings of some legal authorities, there may be limitations placed on my ability to rely on my recollections after hypnosis for purposes of litigation. For example, there is a possibility that anything I remember once hypnosis begins, may not be admissible in a court of law. I acknowledge that __[therapists's name]__ has advised me that if I have any concerns about the legal consequences of hypnosis, that I should consult with my own attorney prior to the use of hypnosis. I hereby agree, freely and voluntarily, to undergo hypnosis. I further agree to release and hold harmless __[therapist's name]__ from any claims or liabilities arising from the use of or inability to use my recollections, the therapist's notes, audiotapes or videotapes of therapy sessions, or any other limitations on my or the therapist's testimony in a courtroom or forensic setting. In consenting to hypnosis, I hereby agree that I do not have a cause of action against __[therapist's name]__ based on his/her professional and competent use of hypnosis with me.

____
Signed

____
Date

APPENDIX B

SAMPLE INFORMED CONSENT FOR FORENSIC HYPNOSIS INTERVIEWS
CONSENT FOR HYPNOSIS

DATE: ______________________________

TIME: ______________________________

I, ____, hereby agree voluntarily and freely, to undergo hypnosis and be interviewed under hypnosis in order to assist with an investigation. I understand that videotape and audiotape recordings will be made of the entire interview and that these methods of preservation of the interview may be used, as to be determined by my attorneys, for any lawful purpose connected with this investigation. In many jurisdictions, courts have held that a person who has been hypnotized cannot testify in court about anything remembered during or after the hypnosis, except in their own behalf. Consequently, in consenting to hypnosis, I understand there is a possibility that anything remembered, once the hypnosis begins, may not be admissible in a court of law. The only way to fully protect my potential right to testify is to forego the use of hypnosis. I understand that the procedural guidelines courts require in hypnosis situations will be followed. But, I have had the opportunity to consult with legal counsel concerning my rights, and in consenting to hypnosis, I hereby agree that I do not have a cause of action against [mental health professional's name].

It has been explained to me that memory is imperfect, whether or not hypnosis is used. Memory is not like a tape recorder, and rarely will all the details of any recollection be fully accurate. People have been shown to be capable of filling in gaps in memory, of distorting information, and of being influenced in what is "remembered" by leading questions or suggestions. Our memories may sometimes be influenced through reading, movies, TV, or conversations. Thus, research has shown that there is no guarantee that information remembered through hypnosis (or through ordinary recall) is factually accurate. On the other hand, information that is so remembered through hypnosis may in fact be accurate. But, the only way one may know definitively whether something recalled under hypnosis is accurate is to obtain independent corroboration. Thus, if I should remember something under hypnosis, I should regard this information as simply one more source of data that cannot be relied on as more accurate or necessarily superior to material already in conscious awareness, without corroboration.

____, a mental health professional, has explained the procedures to be used during the course of this hypnosis session and any questions I had concerning this procedure have been answered to my satisfaction. The purpose of this interview under hypnosis is to assist my memory in recalling ____

____

____

____

____

____

____
Interviewee

Witnesses:

____
Mental Health Professional

____
Witness

APPENDIX C

FORENSIC HYPNOTIC INTERVIEW OUTLINE AND CHECKLIST

I. Preparation of setting.

A. Preferably conducted in a quiet setting, free of interruptions, with a comfortable, high-backed chair for the interviewee.

B. TV equipment set up and fully functioning (cameras, recorder, monitor, time-period generator, 3 working microphones, and simultaneous audio recording).

C. Sufficient supply of videotapes and audiotapes.

D. Consent form(s) on hand.

E. Clipboard etc., if needed for automatic writing.

F. Chaperon for interviewees of the opposite sex of the interviewer.

G. Photo line up, identi-kit and/or artist materials.

H. Prepare TV operator to signal about five minutes before tape needs to be changed.

I. In the event that a law enforcement investigator is not used for the interview, then the mental health professional will assume all duties of the law enforcement investigator.

II. The Interview

A. *Law Enforcement Investigator [in a team approach, or otherwise the Mental Health Professional]:*

Opens the interview.

Place

Date

Time

Identifies persons present in the room.

Requests and receives permission from interviewee to record the entire proceedings on videotape.

States purpose of the interview.

[In a team approach, turns the interview over to the mental health professional.]

B. *Mental Health Professional*

1. Establishes rapport and performs mental status examination and evaluation.

2. Explains hypnosis (which may include):

Asks the interviewee if he/she has been previously hypnotized.

Asks what the interviewee knows/has heard about hypnosis.

Defines hypnosis and explains misconceptions, including a discussion that memory is imperfect, in or out of hypnosis.

Describes characteristics or experiential qualities of hypnosis.

3. Describes possible procedures to be used (which may include):

Trance induction and deepening

Time distortion

Mentions potential risks, e.g., reexperiencing of emotions associated with the event.

Inquiry techniques

Mentions that law enforcement investigator will assist in questioning when this is to be part of the interview.

Posthypnotic suggestion

Suggestibility tests or the elicitation of phenomena in a preliminary trance evaluation and during hypnotic interview.

4. Administers any informal or standardized measures of hypnotic responsivity that are to be used.

Returns attention to the law enforcement investigator when a team approach is used.

C. *Law Enforcement Investigator [in a team approach, or otherwise the Mental Health Professional]:*

Obtains informed consent.

Asks interviewee to describe the event in question. This is a detailed recounting, allowing the interviewee to review the event as he/she pleases. Do not question the interviewee.

Turns the attention to the mental health professional when a team approach is being used.

D. *Mental Health Professional*

Conducts hypnotic induction for the interview, eliciting any hypnotic phenomena deemed desirable to demonstrate hypnotic capacity, whether or not a formal measure was used.

Facilitates age/time regression.

E. *Law Enforcement Investigator [in a team approach, or otherwise the Mental Health Professional]:*

Allows free recall with minimal non-leading questioning concerning the content of the memory, simple repetition of patient phrases verbatim, or comments (e.g., "Um-hmm," "Yes," "Go on," "What are you aware of?") that simply encourage the interviewee to continue.

Conducts non-leading inquiry (use the present tense). If descriptions are obtained in hypnosis, have the interviewee report them again following the termination of hypnosis. A posthypnotic suggestion by the mental health professional may assist in providing recall of the descriptions out of hypnosis.

The mental health professional may deal with emotionality and deepen the hypnosis as needed.

Returns attention to the mental health professional when using a team approach.

F. *Mental Health Professional*

Termination of hypnosis.

Before stopping the videotaping, ask the interviewee, "How do you feel?" Do not stop the taping until the interviewee indicates that she/he is okay.

Breaks may be needed to change tape, use the lavatory, or possibly allow for meals. Hypnosis should be terminated before breaks, and on tape a precautionary statement made that the case is not to be discussed.

In a team approach, the mental health professional is responsible for terminating or re-initiating hypnosis as needed.

The mental health professional should dictate a short statement at the conclusion of the interview to detail the procedure utilized and his/her observations during the session (e.g., depth of trance, phenomena elicited, hypnotizability score), and his/her opinion regarding the validity of the hypnotic state. This note should be maintained with the case file and a copy kept by the mental health professional.

REFERENCES

Agosta, C., & Loring, H. (1988). Understanding and treating the adult retrospective victim of child sexual abuse. Chapter in S. M. Sgroi (Ed.), *Vulnerable Populations* (Vol. 1). Lexington, MA: Lexington Books.

American Medical Association, Council on Scientific Affairs. (1985). Scientific status of refreshing recollection by the use of hypnosis. *Journal of the American Medical Association, 253,* 1918-1923.

American Medical Association, Council on Scientific Affairs. (1994). Memories of childhood abuse. CSA Report 5-A-94.

American Psychiatric Association. (1994). Statement on memories of sexual abuse. Washington, D.C.: APA.

Ault, R. L. (1979). FBI guidelines for use of hypnosis. *International Journal of Clinical & Experimental Hypnosis, 27,* 449-451.

Ault, R. L. (1980). Hypnosis: The FBI's team approach. *FBI Law Enforcement Bulletin,* January, 1980, 1-2.

Archibald, H. C., & Tuddenham, R. D. (1965). Persistent stress reaction after combat. *Archives of General Psychiatry, 12,* 475-481.

Baker, R. A. (1982). The effect of suggestion on past-lives regression. *American Journal of Clinical Hypnosis, 25*(1), 71-76.

Barnier, A. J., & McConkey, K. M. (1992). Reports of real and false memories: The relevance of hypnosis, hypnotizability, and context of memory test. *Journal of Abnormal Psychology, 101*(3), 521-527.

Bartlett, F. C. (1932). *Remembering.* Cambridge: Cambridge University Press.

Beahrs, J. O. (1988). Hypnosis cannot be fully nor reliably excluded from the courtroom. *American Journal of Clinical Hypnosis, 31,* 18-27.

Bekerian, D. A., & Bowers, J. M. (1983). Eyewitness testimony: Were we mislead? *Journal of Experimental Psychology: Learning, Memory & Cognition, 9,* 139-145.

Bennett, H. L. (1988). Perception and memory for events during adequate general anesthesia for surgical operations. Chapter in H. M. Pettinati (Ed.), *Hypnosis & Memory.* New York: Guilford, pp. 193-231.

Berliner, L., & Wheeler, J. R. (1987). Treating the effects of sexual abuse on children. *Journal of Interpersonal Violence, 2,* 415-434.

Bernstein, E., & Putnam, F. W. (1986). Development, reliability and validity of a dissociation scale. *Journal of Nervous & Mental Disease, 174,* 727-735.

Blake-White, J., & Kline, C. M. (1985). Treating the dissociative process in adult victims of childhood incest. *Social Casework, 66,* 394-402.

Blaney, P. H. (1986). Affect and memory: A review. *Psychological Bulletin, 99*(2), 229-246.

Block, E. (1976). *Hypnosis: A New Tool in Crime Detection.* New York: David McKay.

Bohannon, J. N. (1990). Arousal and memory: Quantity and consistency over the years. Paper presented at the Conference on Affect and Flashbulb Memories, Emory University.

Bower, G. H. (1981). Mood and memory. *American Psychologist, 36,* 129-148.

Bowers, J. M., & Bekerian, D. A. (1984). When will postevent information distort eyewitness testimony? *Journal of Applied Psychology, 69,* 466-472.

Bowers, K. (1976). *Hypnosis for the Seriously Curious.* Monterey: Brooks/Cole.

Bowers, K. S., & Davidson, T. M. (1991). A neodissociative critique Spanos's social-psychological model of hypnosis. Chapter in S. J. Lynn & J. W. Rhue (Eds.), *Theories of Hypnosis.* New York: Guilford, pp. 105-143.

Bremner, J. D., Scott, T. M., Delaney, R. C., Southwick, S. M., Mason, J. W., Johnson, D. R., Innis, R. B., McCarthy, G., & Charney, D. S. (1993). Deficits in short-term memory in PTSD. *American Journal of Psychiatry, 150,* 1015-1019.

Brewin, C., Andrews, B. , & Gotlib, I. (1993). Psychopathology and early experience: A reappraisal of retrospective reports. *Psychological Bulletin, 113,* 82-98.

Briere, J., & Conte, J. (1993). Self-reported amnesia for abuse in adults molested as children. *Journal of Traumatic Stress, 6*(1), 21-31.

Brown, D. (1995). Pseudomemories, the standard of science, and the standard of care in trauma treatment. *American Journal of Clinical Hypnosis, 37*(3), 1-24.

Brown, W. (1918). The treatment of cases of shell shock in an advanced neurological centre. *Lancet,* (August 17), 197-200.

Brown, W. (1919). Hypnosis, suggestion, and dissociation. *British Medical Journal, 191,* 734-736.

Brown, W. (1920-1921). The revival of emotional memories and its therapeutic value. *British Journal of Medical Psychology, 1,* 16-19.

Bruck, M., Ceci, S. J., Francouer, E., & Barr, R. (in press). "I hardly cried when I got my shots!" Influencing children's reports about a visit to their pediatrician. *Child Development.*

Burkett, E., & Bruni, F. (1993). *A Gospel of Shame.* New York: Viking.

Cahill, L., Prins, B., Weber, M., & McGaugh, J. L. (1994). B-adrenergic activation and memory for emotional events. *Nature, 371* (Oct. 20, 1994), 702-704.

Cavenar, J. O., & Nash, J. L. (1976). The effects of combat on the normal personality: War neurosis in Vietnam returnees. *Comprehensive Psychiatry, 17,* 647-653.

Cheek, D., & LeCron, L. (1968). *Clinical Hypnotherapy.* New York: Grune & Stratton.

Christiaansen, R. E., & Ochalek, K. (1983). Editing misleading information from memory: Evidence for the coexistence of original and postevent information. *Memory and Cognition, 11,* 467-475.

Christianson, S-A (1984). The relationship between induced emotional arousal and amnesia. *Scandinavian Journal of Psychology, 25,* 147-160.

Christianson, S-A. (1992a). Remembering emotional events: Potential mechanisms. Chapter in S-A Christianson (Ed.), *Handbook of Emotion and Memory.* Hillsdale, N.J.: Laurence Erlbaum, pp. 307-340.

Christianson, S-A. (1992b). Emotional stress and eyewitness memory: A critical review. *Psychological Bulletin, 112*(2), 284-309.

Christianson, S-A. (Ed.) (1992c). *Handbook of Emotion and Memory.* Hillsdale, N.J.: Laurence Erlbaum.

Christianson, S-A. (1992d). Emotional memories in laboratory studies versus real-life studies: Do they compare? Chapter in M. A. Conway, D. C. Rubin, H. Spinnler, & W. A. Wagenaar (Eds.), *Theoretical Perspectives on Autobiographical Memory.* Dordrecht: Kluwer Academic Publishers, pp. 339-352.

Christianson, S.-A., & Hubinette, B. (1993). Hands up! A study of witnesses' emotional reactions and memories associated with bank robberies. *Applied Cognitive Psychology, 7,* 365-379.

Christianson, S.-A. (1994, July 25). Personal communication.

Clifford, B. R., & Hollin, C. R. (1981). Effect of the type of incident and the number of perpetrators on eyewitness memory. *Journal of Applied Psychology, 66,* 364-370.

Clifford, B. R., & Scott, J. (1978). Individual and situational factors in eyewitness testimony. *Journal of Applied Psychology, 63,* 352-359.

Coe, W. C., & Sarbin, T. R. (1991). Role theory: Hypnosis from a dramaturgical and narrational perspective. Chapter in S. J. Lynn & J. W. Rhue (Eds.), *Theories of Hypnosis.* New York: Guilford, pp. 303-323.

Coons, P. M. (1980). Multiple personality: Diagnostic considerations. *Journal of Clinical Psychiatry, 41,* 330-336.

Coons, P. M. (1992). Psychogenic amnesia: A clinical investigation of 25 cases. *Dissociation, 5*(2), 73-79.

Coons, P. M., & Milstein, V. (1990). Self-mutilation associated with dissociative disorders. *Dissociation, 3*(2), 81-87.

Council, J., Kirsch, I., Vickery, A. R., & Carlson, D. (1983). "Trance" vs. "skill" hypnotic inductions: The effects of credibility, expectancy, and experimenter modeling. *Journal of Consulting & Clinical Psychology, 51,* 432-440.

Council, J. R., Kirsch, I., & Hafner, L. P. (1986). Expectancy versus absorption in the prediction of hypnotic responding. *Journal of Personality & Social Psychology, 50,* 182-189.

Crasilneck, H. B., & Hall, J. (1985). *Clinical Hypnosis: Principles & Applications* (Second Edition). Boston: Allyn & Bacon.

Crasilneck, H. B., McCranie, E. J., & Jenkins, M. T. (1956). Special indications for hypnosis as a method of anesthesia. *Journal of the American Medical Association, 162,* 1606-1608.

Crawford, H. J., & Allen, S. N. (1983). Enhanced visual memory during hypnosis as mediated by hypnotic responsiveness and cognitive strategies. *Journal of Experimental Psychology: General, 112,* 662-685.

Crawford, H. J., & Gruzelier, J. H. (1992). A midstream view of the neuropsychophysiology of hypnosis: Recent research and future directions. Chapter in E. Fromm and M. R. Nash (Eds.), *Contemporary Hypnosis Research.* New York: Guilford, pp. 227-266.

Cutshall, J. L., & Yuille, J. C. (1989). Field studies of eyewitness memory of actual crimes. In D. C. Raskin (Ed.), *Psychological Methods in Criminal Investigation and Evidence.* New York: Springer, pp. 97-124.

Daubert v. Merrell Dow Pharmaceuticals, Ind. (1993). 125 L.Ed. 2d 469.

DeBenedittis, G., & Sironi, V. A. (1986). Depth cerebral electrical activity in man during hypnosis. *International Journal of Clinical & Experimental Hypnosis, 34,* 63-70.

DeBenedittis, G., & Sironi, V. A. (1988). Arousal effects of electrical deep brain stimulation in hypnosis. *International Journal of Clinical & Experimental Hypnosis, 36*(2), 96-106.

De Pascalis, V., & Penna, P. M. (1990). 40-Hz EEG activity during hypnotic induction and hypnotic testing. *International Journal of Clinical & Experimental Hypnosis, 38,* 125-138.

Diamond, B. L. (1980). Inherent problems in the use of pretrial hypnosis on a prospective witness. *California Law Review, 68,* 313-349.

Dutton, D. G. (1986). Wife assaulters' explanations for assault: The neutralization of self-punishment. *Canadian Journal of Behavioral Science, 18,* 381-390.

Dywan, J., & Bowers, K. (1983). The use of hypnosis to enhance recall. *Science, 222,* 184-185.

El-Rayes, M. (1982). Traumatic war neurosis: Egyptian experience. *Journal of the Royal Army Medical Corps, 128,* 67-71.

Erdelyi, M. H. (1985). *Psychoanalysis: Freud's Cognitive Psychology.* New York: W. H. Freeman.

Erdelyi, M. H. (1988). Hypermnesia: The effect of hypnosis, fantasy, and concentration. Chapter in H. M. Pettinati (Ed.), *Hypnosis & Memory.* New York: Guilford, pp. 64-94.

Erdelyi, M. H. (1994). Hypnotic hypermnesia: The empty set of hypermnesia. *International Journal of Clinical & Experimental Hypnosis, 42*(4), 379-390.

Erickson, M. H. (1980). *The Collected Papers of Milton H. Erickson, M.D.. Volumes 1-4.* Edited by E. L. Rossi. New York: Irvington.

Eth, S., & Pynoos, R. S. (Eds.) (1985). *Post Traumatic Stress Disorders in Children.* Washington: American Psychoanalytic Association.

Feldman-Summers, S., & Pope, K. S. (1994). The experience of "forgetting" childhood abuse: A national survey of psychologists. *Journal of Consulting & Clinical Psychology, 62*(3), 636-639.

Fisher, C. (1943). Hypnosis in treatment of neuroses due to war and to other causes. *War Medicine, 4,* 565-576.

Fisher, C. (1945). Amnesic states in war neurosis: The psychogenesis of fugue. *Psychoanalytic Quarterly, 14,* 437-468.

Fisher, R. P., Geiselman, R. E., & Amador, M. (1989). Field test of the cognitive interview: Enhancing the recollection of actual victims and witnesses of crime. *Journal of Applied Psychology, 74*(5), 722-727.

Frankel, F. H. (1975). Physical symptoms and marked hypnotizability. *International Journal of Clinical & Experimental Hypnosis, 23*(4), 227-233.

Frankel, F. H. (1988). The clinical use of hypnosis in aiding recall. Chapter in H. Pettinati (Ed.), *Hypnosis and Memory.* New York: Guilford, pp. 247-264.

Frankel, F. H. (1994). Personal correspondence to D. Corydon Hammond. July 1, 1994.

Freyd, J. J. (1994). Betrayal-trauma: Traumatic amnesia as an adaptive response to childhood abuse. *Ethics & Behavior, 4*(4), in press.

Frischholz, E. J., Lipman, L. S., Braun, B. G., & Sachs, R. G. (1992). Psychopathology, hypnotizability, and dissociation. *American Journal of Psychiatry, 149*(11), 1521-1525.

Fromm, E. (1992). An ego-psychological theory of hypnosis. Chapter in E. Fromm and M. R. Nash (Eds.), *Contemporary Hypnosis Research.* New York: Guilford, pp. 131-148.

Frye v. United States (1923). 54 App. D.C. 46, 293 F. 1013.

Garry, M., & Loftus, E. F. (1994). Pseudomemories without hypnosis. *International Journal of Clinical & Experimental Hypnosis 42*(4), 363-378.

Garver, R. B. (1987). Investigative hypnosis. Chapter in W. C. Wester Ed.), *Clinical Hypnosis: A Case Management Approach.* Cincinnati: Behavioral Science Center, pp. 213-225.

Geiselman, R. E., Fisher, R. P., MacKinnon, D. P., & Holland, H. L. (1985). Eyewitness memory enhancement in the police interview: Cognitive retrieval mnemonics versus hypnosis. *Journal of Applied Psychology, 70,* 401-412.

Geiselman, R. E., & Machlovitz, H. (1987). Hypnosis memory recall: Implications for forensic use. *American Journal of Forensic Psychology, 1,* 37-47.

Gelinas, D. J. (1983). The persisting negative effects of incest. *Psychiatry, 46,* 312-332.

Gerlsma, C., Emmelkamp, P. M. G., Arrindell, W. A. (1990). Anxiety, depression, and perception of early parenting: A metaanalysis. *Clinical Psychology Review, 10,* 251-277.

Goldfeld, A. E., Mollica, R. F., Pesavento, B. H. et al. (1988). The physical and psychological sequelae of torture: Symptomatology and diagnosis. *Journal of the American Medical Association, 259,* 2725-2729.

Goodman, G. S., Hirschman, J. E., Hepps, D., & Rudy, L. (1991). Children's memory for stressful events. *Merrill Palmer Quarterly, 37,* 109-158.

Gravitz, M. A. (1993). Etienne Felix d'Henin de Cuvillers: A founder of hypnosis. *American Journal of Clinical Hypnosis, 36*(1), 7-11.

Grinker, R. R., & Spiegel, J. P. (1945). *Men Under Stress.* Philadelphia: Blakiston.

Grinker, R. R., & Spiegel, J. P. (1943). *War Neuroses in North Africa.* New York: Josiah Macy, Jr. Foundation.

Gudjonsson, G. H. (1984). A new scale of interrogative suggestibility. *Personality & Individual Differences, 5*(3), 303-314.

Gudjonsson, G. (1992). *The Psychology of Interrogations, Confessions and Testimony.* New York: John Wiley & Sons.

Halverson, C. F. (1988). Remembering your parents: Reflections on the retrospective method. *Journal of Personality, 56,* 435-443.

Hammond, D. C. (1990). (Ed.). *Handbook of Hypnotic Suggestions and Metaphors.* New York: W. W. Norton.

Hammond, D. C. (1994). *Medical and Psychological Hypnosis: How It Benefits Patients.* Des Plaines, IL: American Society of Clinical Hypnosis Press.

Hammond , D. C. & Elkins G. R. (1994). *Standards of Training in Clinical Hypnosis.* Des Plaines, IL: American Society of Clinical Hypnosis.

Henderson, J. L., & Moore, M. (1944). The psychoneuroses of war. New *England Journal of Medicine, 230,* 273-279.

Hendin, H., Hass, A. P., Singer, P., et al. (1984). The reliving experience in Vietnam veterans with posttraumatic stress disorder. *Comprehensive Psychiatry, 25,* 165-173.

Herman, J. L. (1985). Histories of violence in an outpatient population: An exploratory study. *American Journal of Orthopsychiatry, 55.*

Herman, J. L., & Schatzow, E. (1987). Recovery and verification of memories of childhood sexual trauma. *Psychoanalytic Psychology, 4,* 1-14.

Heuer, F., & Reisberg, D. (1990). Vivid memories of emotional events: The accuracy of remembered minutiae. *Memory & Cognition, 18,* 496-506.

Heuer, F., & Reisberg, D. (1992). Emotion, arousal, and memory for detail. Chapter in S-A Christianson (Ed.), *The Handbook of Emotion and Memory.* Hillsdale, N.J.: Lawrence Erlbaum, pp. 151-180.

Hibler, N. S. (1984). Forensic hypnosis: To hypnotize, or not to hypnotize, that is the question! *American Journal of Clinical Hypnosis, 27*(1), 52-57.

Hilgard, E. R. (1965). *Hypnotic Susceptibility.* New York: Harcourt, Brace, Jovanovich.

Hilgard, E. R. (1978). States of consciousness in hypnosis: Divisions or levels? Chapter in F. H. Frankel and H. S. Zamansky (Eds.), *Hypnosis at its Bicentennial: Selected Papers*. New York: Plenum, pp. 15-36.

Hilgard, E. R. (1977, 1986). *Divided Consciousness: Multiple Controls in Human Thought and Action*. New York: Wiley-Interscience.

Hilgard, E. R. (1992). Dissociation and theories of hypnosis. Chapter in E. Fromm and M. R. Nash (Eds.), *Contemporary Hypnosis Research*. New York: Guilford, pp. 69-101.

Hilgard, E. R., & Hilgard, J. R. (1983). *Hypnosis in the Relief of Pain* (Revised Edition). Los Altos, CA: William Kaufmann, Inc.

Hilgard, J. R. (1970). *Personality and Hypnosis*. Chicago: University of Chicago Press.

Horowitz, M. J., & Reidbord, S. P. (1992). Memory, emotion, and response to trauma. Chapter in S.-A. Christianson (Ed.), *The Handbook of Emotion and Memory: Research & Theory*. Hillsdale, N.J.: Lawrence Erlbaum, pp. 343-358.

Horowitz, M. J., Wilner, N., Kaltreider, N., & Alvarez, W. (1980). Signs and symptoms of post-traumatic stress disorder. *Archives of General Psychiatry, 37,* 85-92.

Hull, C. L. (1933). *Hypnosis and Suggestibility: An Experimental Approach*. New York: Appleton-Century Crofts.

Jaffe, R. (1968). Dissociative phenomena in former concentration camp inmates. *International Journal of Psychoanalysis, 49,* 310-312.

Johnston, J. C., Chajkowaski, J., DuBreuil, S. C., & Spanos, N. P. (1989). The effects of manipulated expectancies on behavioural and subjective indices of hypnotisability. *Australian Journal of Clinical & Experimental Hypnosis, 17,* 121-130.

Jones, D. P. H., & Krugman, R. D. (1986). Can a three-year-old child bear witness to her sexual assault and attempted murder? *Child Abuse & Neglect, 10,* 253-258.

Kalman, G. (1977). On combat neurosis: Psychiatric experience during the recent Middle East war. *International Journal of Social Psychiatry, 23,* 195-203.

Kanovitz, J. (1992). Hypnotic memories and civil sexual abuse trials. *Vanderbilt Law Review, 45,* 1185-1262.

Kardiner, A. (1941). *The Traumatic Neuroses of War*. New York: Hoeber.

Kardiner, A., & Spiegel, H. (1947). *War, Stress, and Neurotic Illness*. New York: Hoeber.

Kaszniak. A. W., Nussbaum, P. D., Berren, M. R., et al., (1988). Amnesia as a consequence of male rape: A case report. *Journal of Abnormal Psychology, 97,* 100-104.

Kihlstrom, J. (1994). Hypnosis, delayed recall, and the principles of memory. *International Journal of Clinical & Experimental Hypnosis, 42*(4), 337-345.

Kinzie, J. D. (1993). Posttraumatic effects and their treatment among Southeast Asian refugees. Chapter in J. P. Wilson & B. Raphael (Eds.), *International Handbook of Traumatic Stress Syndromes.* New York: London, pp. 311-319.

Kirsch, I. (1991). The social learning theory of hypnosis. Chapter in S. J. Lynn & J. Rhue (Eds.), *Theories of Hypnosis: Current Models and Perspectives.* New York: Guilford, pp. 439-466.

Kirsch, I., Council, J. R., & Mobayed, C. (1987). Imagery and response expectancy as determinants of hypnotic behavior. *British Journal of Experimental & Clinical Hypnosis, 4,* 25-31.

Kline, M. V. (1958). *Freud and Hypnosis.* New York: Julian Press and The Institute for Research in Hypnosis.

Kluft, R. P. (1990). The fractionated abreaction technique. In D. C. Hammond (Ed.), *Handbook of Hypnotic Suggestions & Metaphors.* New York: W. W. Norton, pp. 527-528.

Kolb, L. C. (1985). The place of narcosynthesis in the treatment of chronic and delayed stress reactions of war. Chapter in S. M. Sonnenberg, A. S. Blank, & J. A. Talbott (Eds.), *The Trauma of War: Stress and Recovery in Viet Nam Veterans.* Washington, DC: American Psychiatric Association Press, 211-226.

Kroger, W. S., & Douce, R. G. (1979). Hypnosis in criminal investigation. *International Journal of Clinical & Experimental Hypnosis, 27,* 358-374.

Krystal, H. (1993). Beyond the DSM-III-R: Therapeutic considerations in posttraumatic stress disorder. Chapter in J. P. Wilson and B. Raphael (Eds.), *International Handbook of Traumatic Stress Syndromes.* New York: Plenum, pp. 841-854.

Kubie, L. S. (1943). Manual of emergency treatment for acute war neuroses. *War Medicine, 4,* 582-599.

Kuehn, L. L. (1974). Looking down a gun barrel: Person perception and violent crime. *Perceptual & Motor Skills, 39,* 1159-1164.

Labelle, L., Laurence, J.-R., Nadon, R., & Perry, C. (1990). Hypnotizability, preference for an imagic cognitive style, and memory creation in hypnosis. *Journal of Abnormal Psychology, 99,* 222-228.

Lanning, K. (1994). Personal communication to Alan Scheflin, Sixth Annual Eastern Regional Conference on Abuse and Multiple Personality, Alexandria, Virginia, June, 1994.

Laurence, J.-R. (1982). Memory creation in hypnosis. Unpublished doctoral dissertation, Concordia University, Montreal, Canada.

Laurence, J.-R., & Perry, C. (1983). Hypnotically created memory among high hypnotizable subjects. *Science, 222,* 523-524.

LeDoux, J. E. (1992). Emotion as memory: Anatomical systems underlying indelible neural traces. Chapter in S-A Christianson (Ed.), *Handbook of Emotion and Memory*. Hillsdale, N.J.: Laurence Erlbaum, pp. 269-288.

LeDoux, J. E. (1994). Emotion, memory and the brain. *Scientific American, 270*(6), 50-57.

Leippe, M. R. (1980). Effects of integrative memorial and cognitive processes on the correspondence of accuracy and confidence. *Law and Human Behavior, 4,* 261-274.

Lewinsohn, P. M., & Rosenbaum, M. (1987). Recall of parental behavior by acute depressives, remitted depressives and nondepressives. *Journal of Personality & Social Psychology, 52,* 611-619.

Lieberman, M. A., Yalom, E. D., & Miles, M. B. (1973). *Encounter Groups: First Facts.* New York: Basic Books.

Loewenstein, R. J. (1991). Psychogenic amnesia and psychogenic fugue: A comprehensive review. Chapter in A. Tasmann & S. M. Goldfinger, *American Psychiatric Press Review of Psychiatry, Vol. 10.* Washington, DC: American Psychiatric Press, 189-221.

Loftus, E. F. (1979). *Eyewitness Testimony.* Cambridge, MA: Harvard University Press.

Loftus, E. F. (1993). The reality of repressed memories. *American Psychologist, 48*(5), 518-537.

Loftus, E. F., & Burns, T. (1982). Mental shock can produce retrograde amnesia. *Memory & Cognition, 10,* 318-323.

Loftus, E. F., & Coan, J. (in press). The construction of childhood memories. Chapter in D. P. Peters (Ed.), *The Child Witness in Context: Cognitive. Social. and Legal Perspectives.* Dordrecht, Netherlands: Kluwer.

Loftus, E. F., & Palmer, J. C. (1974). Reconstruction of automobile destruction: An example of the interaction between language and memory. *Journal of Verbal Learning and Verbal Behavior, 13,* 585-589.

Loftus, E. F., Polonsky, S., & Fullilove, M. T. (1994). Memories of childhood sexual abuse: Remembering and repressing. *Psychology of Women Quarterly, 18,* 67-84.

Loftus, E. F., & Zanni, G. (1975). Eyewitness testimony: The influence of the wording of a question. *Bulletin of the Psychonomic Society, 5,* 86-88.

Lynn, S. J., Milano, M., & Weekes, J. R. (1991). Hypnosis and pseudomemories: The effects of prehypnotic expectancies. *Journal of Personality & Social Psychology, 60,* 318-326.

Lynn, S. J., Milano, M., & Weekes, J. R. (1992). Pseudomemory and age regression: An exploratory study. *American Journal of Clinical Hypnosis, 35*(2), 129-137.

Lynn, S. J., & Rhue, J. (Ed.) (1991). *Theories of Hypnosis.* New York: Guilford.

Lynn, S. J., Rhue, J. W., Myers, B. P., & Weekes, J. R. (1994). Pseudomemory in hypnotized and simulating subjects. *International Journal of Clinical & Experimental Hypnosis, 42*(2), 118-129.

Lynn, S. J., Weekes, J. R., & Milano, M. J. (1989). Reality versus suggestion: Pseudomemory in hypnotizable and simulating subjects. *Journal of Abnormal Psychology, 98,* 137-144.

Madakasira, S., & O'Brien,K. (1987). Acute posttraumatic stress disorder in victims of a natural disaster. *Journal of Nervous & Mental Disease, 175,* 286-290.

Maltz, W. (1988). Identifying and treating sexual repercussions of incest: A couples therapy approach. *Journal of Sex & Marital Therapy, 14,* 145-163.

McCann, T., & Sheehan, P. W. (1987). The breaching of pseudomemory under hypnotic instruction: Implications for original memory retrieval. *British Journal of Experimental & Clinical Hypnosis, 4,* 101-108.

McCann, T., & Sheehan, P. W., (1988). Hypnotically induced pseudomemories —sampling their conditions among hypnotizable subjects. *Journal of Personality & Social Psychology, 54,* 239-246.

McCann, T., & Sheehan, P. W. (1989). Pseudomemory creation and confidence in the experimental hypnosis context. *British Journal of Experimental & Clinical Hypnosis, 6*(3), 151-159.

McCloskey, M., & Zaragoza, M. (1985). Misleading postevent information and memory for events: Arguments and evidence against memory impairment hypotheses. *Journal of Experimental Psychology, 114*(1), 1-16.

McConkey, K. M. (1992). The effects of hypnotic procedures on remembering: The experimental findings and their implications for forensic hypnosis. Chapter in E. Fromm & M. R. Nash (Eds.), *Contemporary Hypnosis Research.* New York: Guilford, pp. 405-426.

McConkey, K. M., & Jupp, J. J. (1985). Opinions about the forensic use of hypnosis. *Australian Psychologist, 20,* 283-291.

McConkey, K. M., Labelle, L., Bibb, B. C., & Bryant, R. A. (1990). Hypnosis and suggested pseudomemory: The relevance of test context. *Australian Journal of Psychology, 42,* 197-205.

McConkey, K. M., Roche, S. M., & Sheehan, P. W. (1989). Reports of forensic hypnosis: A critical analysis. *Australian Psychologist, 24,* 249-272.

McDougall, W. (1920-1921). The revival of emotional memories and its therapeutic value (III). *British Journal of Medical Psychology, 1,* 23-29.

McGaugh, J. L. (1992). Affect, neuromodulatory systems, and memory storage. Chapter in S-A Christianson (Ed.), *Handbook of Emotion and Memory.* Hillsdale, N.J.: Laurence Erlbaum, pp. 245-268.

Meares, A. (1961). *A System of Medical Hypnosis.* Philadelphia: Saunders.

Mingay, D. J. (1986). Hypnosis and memory for incidentally learned scenes. *British Journal of Experimental & Clinical Hypnosis, 3,* 173-183.

Munsterberg, H. (1908). *On the Witness Stand.* New York: Doubleday, Page, & Company.

Murrey, G. J., Cross, H. J., & Whipple, J. (1992). Hypnotically created pseudomemories: Further investigation into the "memory distortion or response bias" question. *Journal of Abnormal Psychology, 101*(1), 75-77.

Mutter, C. B. (1984). The use of hypnosis with defendants. *American Journal of Clinical Hypnosis, 27*(1), 42-51.

Mutter, C. B. (1990). Hypnosis with defendants: Does it really work? *American Journal of Clinical Hypnosis, 32*(4), 257-262.

Myers, C. S. (1915). A contribution to the study of shell-shock. *Lancet,* (February 13), 316-320.

Myers, C. S. (1916). Contributions to the study of shell-shock. *Lancet,* (January 8), 65-69.

Nash, M. R. (1994). Memory distortion and sexual trauma: The problem of false negatives and false positives. *International Journal of Clinical & Experimental Hypnosis 42*(4), 346-362.

Neisser, U., & Harsch, N. (1990, February). Phantom flashbulbs: False recollections of hearing the news about Challenger. Paper presented at the Emory Cognition Project Conference on Affect and Flashbulb Memories, Atlanta, Georgia.

Niederland, W. G. (1968). Clinical observations on the "survivor syndrome." *International Journal of Psychoanalysis, 49,* 313-315.

Nilsson, L-G., & Archer, T. (1992). Biological aspects of memory and emotion: Affect and cognition. Chapter in S-A Christianson (Ed.), *Handbook of Emotion and Memory.* Hillsdale, N.J.: Laurence Erlbaum, pp. 289-306.

Odgers, S. J. (1988). Evidence law and previously hypnotized witnesses. *Australian Journal of Clinical & Experimental Hypnosis, 16,* 91-102.

Orne, M. T. (1977). The construct of hypnosis: Implications of the definition for research and practice. In W. E. Edmonston (Ed.), Conceptual and investigative approaches to hypnosis and hypnotic phenomena. *Annals of the New York Academy of Sciences, 296*(1), 14-33.

Orne, M. T. (1979). The use and misuse of hypnosis in court. *International Journal of Clinical & Experimental Hypnosis, 27,* 311-341.

Ornstein, P. A., Gordon, B. N., & Baker-Ward, L. (in press). Children's memory for salient events: Implications for testimony. Chapter in M. Howe, C. Brainerd, & V. Reyna (Eds.), *Development of Long-Term Retention.* New York: Springer-Verlag.

Ornstein, P. A., Gordon, B. N., Baker-Ward, L. E., & Merrit, K. A. (in press). Chapter in D-P. Peters (Ed.), *The Child Witness in Context: Cognitive, Social, and Legal Perspectives.* Dordrecht, The Netherlands: Kluwer Academic Publishers.

Parfitt, D. N., & Caryle-Gall, C. M. (1944). Psychogenic amnesia: The refusal to remember. *Journal of Mental Science, 379,* 519-531.

People v. Caro, 46 Cal.3d 1194, 255 Cal. Rptr. 569, 767 p.2d 1047 (1988).

People v. Johnson, 47 Cal.3d 1194, 255 Cal. Rptr. 569, 767 P.2d 1047 (1989).

Perry, J. C., & Jacobs, D. (1982). Overview: Clinical applications of the amytal interview in psychiatric emergency settings. *American Journal of Psychiatry, 139,* 552-559.

Pettinati, H. M. (1988). *Hypnosis and Memory.* New York: Guilford.

Piaget, J. (1954). *The Construction of Reality in the Child.* New York: Basic Books.

Pillemer, D. B. (1984). Flashbulb memories of the assassination attempt on President Reagan. *Cognition, 16,* 63-80.

Pitman, R. K. (May, 1994). Hormonal modulation of traumatic memory. Scientific paper presented at the annual meeting of the American Psychiatric Association, Philadelphia, Pennsylvania.

Putnam, W. H. (1979). Hypnosis and distortions in eyewitness memory. *International Journal of Clinical & Experimental Hypnosis, 27,* 437-448.

Rainer, D. (1983). Eyewitness testimony: Does hypnosis enhance accuracy, distortion, and confidence? Unpublished doctoral dissertation, University of Wyoming.

Raginsky, B. B. (1969). Hypnotic recall of aircrash cause. *International Journal of Clinical & Experimental Hypnosis, 17,* 1-19.

Rath, B. (1982). The use of suggestions during general anesthesia. Unpublished doctoral dissertation, University of Louisville.

Read, J. D., Yuille, J. C., & Tollestrup, P. (1992). Recollections of a robbery: Effects of arousal and alcohol and person identification. *Law & Human Behavior.*

Reisberg, D., Heuer, F., Mclean, J., & O'Shaughnessy, M. (1988). The quantity, not quality, of affect predicts memory vividness. *Bulletin of the Psychonomic Society, 26,* 100-103.

Reiser, M. (1986, April). Reader's forum. *Division on Psychological Hypnosis Newsletter.* Washington, D.C.: American Psychological Association, pp. 5-6.

Relinger, H. (1984). Hypnotic hypermnesia: A critical review. *American Journal of Clinical Hypnosis, 26,* 212-225.

Rock v. Arkansas, (1987). 107S.Ct. 2704, 97 L.Ed.2d 37.

Rivers, H. R. (1918). The repression of war experience. *Lancet,* (February 2), 173-177.

Rossi, E. L. (1993). *The Psychobiology of Mind-Body Healing* (Revised Edition). New York: W. W. Norton.

Rossi, E. L., & Cheek, D. B. (1988). *Mind-Body Therapy: Ideodynamic Healing in Hypnosis*. New York: W. W. Norton.

Rudy, L., & Goodman, G. S. (1991). Effects of participation on children's reports: Implications for children's testimony. *Developmental Psychology, 27,* 527-538.

Sanders, G. S., & Simmons, W. L. (1983). Use of hypnosis to enhance eyewitness accuracy: Does it work? *Journal of Applied Psychology, 68,* 70-77.

Sanders, S. (1969). The effect of hypnosis on visual imagery. *Dissertation Abstracts International, 30,* 2936B.

Saporta, J. A., & van der Kolk, B. A. (1992). Psychobiological consequences of severe trauma. Chapter in M. Basoglu (Ed.), *Torture and It's Consequences.* New York: Cambridge University Press, pp. 151-181.

Sargant, W., & Slater, E. (1941). Amnesic syndromes in war. *Proceedings of the Royal Society of Medicine, 34,* 757-764.

Saywitz, K. J., Goodman, G. S., Nicholas, E., & Moan. S. F. (1991). Children's memories of a physical examination involving genital touch: Implications for reports of child sexual abuse. *Journal of Consulting & Clinical Psychology, 59,* 682-691.

Schacter, D. L. (1987). Implicit memory: History and current status. *Journal of Experimental Psychology, Learning, Memory and Cognition, 13,* 501-516.

Schacter, D. L., & Kihlstrom, J.F. (1989). Functional amnesia. Chapter in F. Boller & J.Grafman (Eds.), *Handbook of Neuropsychology.* Amsterdam: Elsevier.

Scheflin, A. W. (1994a). Forensic hypnosis and the law: The current situation in the United States. Chapter in B. J. Evans and R. O. Stanley, *Hypnosis and the Law: Principles and Practices.* Heidelberg, Victoria, Australia: Australian Journal of Clinical & Experimental Hypnosis.

Scheflin, A. W. (1994b). Forensic hypnosis: Unanswered questions. *Australian Journal of Clinical & Experimental Hypnosis, 22*(1), 23-34.

Scheflin, A. W., Brown, D. P., & Hammond, D. C. (1995, in press). *Repressed Memory, Hypnotherapy and the Law.* Des Plaines, IL: American Society of Clinical Hypnosis Press.

Scheflin, A. W., & Shapiro, J. L. (1989). *Trance on Trial.* New York: Guilford.

Schwarz, J. C., Barton-Henry, M. L., & Pruzinsky, T. (1985). Assessing child-rearing behaviors: A comparison of ratings made by mother, father, child, and siblings on the CRPBI. *Child Development, 56,* 462-479.

Sheehan, P. W. (1969). Artificial induction of posthypnotic conflict. *Journal of Abnormal Psychology, 74,* 16-25.

Sheehan, P. W. (1979). Hypnosis and the process of imagination. Chapter in E. Fromm & R. E. Shor (Eds.), *Hypnosis: Developments in Research and New Perspectives* (2nd Edition). New York: Aldine, pp. 381-411.

Sheehan, P. W., Garnett, M., & Robertson, R. (1993). The effects of cue level, hypnotizability, and state instruction on responses to leading questions. *International Journal of Clinical & Experimental Hypnosis, 41*(4), 287-304.

Sheehan, P. W., & Grigg, L. (1985). Hypnosis, memory and the acceptance of an implausible cognitive set. *British Journal of Clinical & Experimental Hypnosis, 3,* 5-12.

Sheehan, P. W., Grigg, L., & McCann, T. (1984). Memory distortion following exposure to false information in hypnosis. *Journal of Abnormal Psychology, 93,* 259-265.

Sheehan, P. W., & McConkey, K. M. (1982). *Hypnosis & Experience: The Exploration of Phenomena & Process.* Hillsdale, N.J.: Lawrence Erlbaum.

Sheehan, P. W., Statham, D., & Jamieson, G. A. (199la). Pseudomemory effects over time in the hypnotic setting. *Journal of Abnormal Psychology, 100,* 39-44.

Sheehan, P. W., Statham, D., & Jamieson, G. A. (199lb). Pseudomemory effects and their relationship to level of susceptibility to hypnosis and state instructions. *Journal of Personality & Social Psychology, 60,* 130-137.

Shor, R. E., & Orne, E. C. (1962). *The Harvard Group Scale of Hypnotic Susceptibility Form A.* Palo Alto: Consulting Psychologists Press.

Shore, J. H., Tatum, E. L., & Vollmer, W. M. (1986). Psychiatric reactions to disaster: The Mount St. Helens experience. *American Journal of Psychiatry, 143,* 590-595.

Silver, S. M., & Kelley, M. D. (1985). Hypnotherapy of PTSD in combat veterans from WWII and Vietnam. Chapter in W. E. Kelley (Ed.), *Post-Traumatic Stress Disorders and the Vietnam Veteran.* New York: Brunner/Mazel, 211-233.

Simmel, E. (1944). War neurosis. Chapter in Landor Lorand (Ed.), *Psychoanalysis Today.* New York: International Universities.

Singer, J. A., & Salovey, P. (1988). Mood and memory: Evaluating the network theory of affect. *Clinical Psychology Review, 8,* 211-251.

Smith, M. C. (1983). Hypnotic memory enhancement of witnesses: Does it work? *Psychological Bulletin, 94,* 387-407.

Smyth, L. D. (1982). Psychopathology as a function of neuroticism and a hypnotically implanted aggressive conflict. *Journal of Personality & Social Psychology, 43*(3), 555-564.

Sommerschield, H., & Reyher, J. (1973). Posthypnotic conflict, repression, and psychopathology. *Journal of Abnormal Psychology, 82*(2), 278-290.

Sonnenberg, S. M., Blank, A. S., & Talbott, J. A. (1985). *The Trauma of War: Stress and Recovery in Viet Nam Veterans.* Washington, DC: American Psychiatric Press.

Southard, E. E. (1919). *Shell-Shock and Other Neuropsychiatric Problems.* Boston: W. W. Leonard.

Spanos, N. P., Brett, P. J., Menary, E. P., & Cross, W. P. (1987). A measure of attitudes toward hypnosis: Relationships with absorption and hypnotic susceptibility. *American Journal of Clinical Hypnosis, 30,* 139-150.

Spanos, N. P., & Chaves, J. F. (Eds.) (1989). *Hypnosis: The Cognitive-Behavioral Perspective.* Buffalo: Prometheus Books

Spanos, N. P., Gwynn, M. I., Comer, S. L., Baltruweit, W. J., & de Groh, M. (1989). Are hypnotically induced pseudomemories resistant to cross-examination? *Law & Human Behavior, 13,* 271-289.

Spanos, N. P., & McLean, J. (1986). Hypnotically created pseudomemories: Memory distortions or reporting biases? *British Journal of Experimental & Clinical Hypnosis, 3,* 155-159.

Spanos, N. P., Menary, E., Gabora, N. J., DuBreuil, S. C., & Dewhirst, B. (199la). Secondary identity enactments during hypnotic past-life regression: A sociocognitive perspective. *Journal of Personality & Social Psychology 61,* 308-320.

Spanos, N. P., Quigley, C. A., Gwynn, M. I., Glatt, R. L., & Perlini, A. H. (199lb). Hypnotic interrogation, pretrial preparation, and witness testimony during direct and cross-examination. *Law and Human Behavior, 15*(6), 639-653.

Spiegel, D. (1981). Vietnam grief work using hypnosis. *American Journal of Clinical Hypnosis, 24,* 33-40.

Spiegel, D. (1987). The Shirley decision: The cure is worse than the disease. In R. W. Rieber (Ed.), *Advances in Forensic Psychology and Psychiatry (Vol. 2).* Norwood, N.J.: Ablex.

Spiegel, D. (1993). Hypnosis in the treatment of posttraumatic stress disorder. Chapter in J. W. Rhue, S. J. Lynn, and I. Kirsch (Eds.), *Handbook of Clinical Hypnosis.* Washington, D.C.: American Psychological Association.

Spiegel, D., Hunt, T., & Dondershine, H. E. (1988). Dissociation and hypnotizability in posttraumatic stress disorder. *American Journal of Psychiatry, 145,* 301-305.

Spiegel, D., & Scheflin, A. W. (1994). Dissociated or fabricated? Psychiatric aspects of repressed memory in criminal and civil cases. *International Journal of Clinical & Experimental Hypnosis, 42*(4), 411-432.

Spiegel, D., & Spiegel, H. (1987). Forensic uses of hypnosis. Chapter in I. B. Weinter & A. K. Hess (Eds)., *Handbook of Forensic Psychology.* New York: Wiley, pp. 490-507.

Spiegel, H. (1963). The spectrum of hypnotic and nonhypnotic phenomena. *American Journal of Clinical Hypnosis, 6,* 1-5.

Spiegel, H. (1974). The grade 5 syndrome: The highly hypnotizable person. *International Journal of Clinical & Experimental Hypnosis, 22,* 303-319.

Spiegel, H. (1980). Hypnosis and evidence: Help or hindrance? *Annals of the New York Academy of Sciences, 347,* 73-85.

Spiegel, H., & Greenleaf, M. (1992). Personality style and hypnotizability: The fix-flex continuum. *Psychiatric Medicine, 10*(1), 13-24.

Spiegel, H., & Spiegel, D. (1978/1987). *Trance and Treatment: Clinical Uses of Hypnosis*. New York: Basic Books. Reprinted in 1987, Washington, D.C.: American Psychiatric Press.

State v. Hurd (1981). 86 N.J. 525, 432 A.2d 86.

Steinberg, M. (1994). *Interviewer's Guide to the Structured Clinical Interview for DSM-IV Dissociative Disorders (SCID-D).* Washington, D.C.: American Psychiatric Press.

Steinberg, M., Cicchetti, D., Buchanan, J., Hall, P., & Rounsaville, B. (1993). Clinical assessment of dissociative symptoms and disorders: The Structured Clinical Interview for DSM-IV Dissociative Disorders (SCID-D). *Dissociation, 6*(1), 3-15.

Stutman, R. K., & Bliss, E. L. (1985). Posttraumatic stress disorder, hypnotizability and imagery. *American Journal of Psychiatry, 142,* 741-743.

Tellegen, A. (1979). On measures and conceptions of hypnosis. *American Journal of Clinical Hypnosis, 21,* 219-236.

Terr, L. (1988). What happens to early memories of trauma? A study of twenty children under age five at the time of documented traumatic events. *Journal of the American Academy of Child & Adolescent Psychiatry, 27,* 96-104.

Terr, L. (1991). Childhood traumas: An outline and overview. *American Journal of Psychiatry, 148,* 10-20.

Thom, D. A., & Fenton, N. (1920). Amnesias in war Cases. *American Journal of Insanity, 76,* 437-448.

Torrie, A. (1944). Psychosomatic casualties in the Middle East. *Lancet, 1,* 139-143.

Tulving, E. (1972). Episodic and semantic memory. Chapter in E. Tulving & W. Donaldson (Eds.), *Organization of Memory*. New York: Academic Press, pp. 381-403.

Tulving, E., & Pearlstone, Z. (1966). Availability and accessibility of information in memory for words. *Journal of Verbal Learning and Verbal Behavior, 5,* 381-391.

Tulving, E., & Thomson, D. M. (1973). Encoding specificity and retrieval processes in episodic memory. *Psychological Review, 80,* 352-373.

Tureen, L. L., & Stein, M. (1949). The base section psychiatric hospital. *Bulletin of the U.S. Army Medical Department, 9*(suppl), 105-137.

United States v. Adams, 581 F.2d 193 (9th Cir. 1978), cert. denied, 439 U.S. 1006 (1978).

United States v. Wade, 388 U.S. 218 (1967).

Van der Kolk, B. A. (1984). *Post-Traumatic Stress Disorder: Psychological & Biological Sequelae.* Washington, D.C.: APA Press.

Van der Kolk, B. A. (1987). *Psychological Trauma.* Washington: APA Press.

Van der Kolk, B. A. (1988). The trauma spectrum: The interaction of biological and social events in the genesis of the trauma response. *Journal of Traumatic Stress, 1*(3), 273-290.

Van der Kolk, B. A., & Saporta, J. (1993). Biological response to psychic trauma. Chapter in J. P. Wilson & B. Raphael (Eds.), *International Handbook of Traumatic Stress Syndromes.* New York: Plenum, pp. 25-34.

Van der Kolk, B. A., & Van der Hart, O. (1991). The intrusive past: The flexibility of memory and the engraving of trauma. *American Imago, 48*(4), 425-454.

Van der Kolk, B. A., Vardi, D. J., Eisler, R. E., Herron, N., Hostettler, A., & Zakai, A. (1994). Traumatic versus autobiographical memory. Scientific paper delivered at the American Psychiatric Association annual meeting, May, 1994, Philadelphia, Pennsylvania.

Wagenaar, W. A., & Groeneweg, J. (1990). The memory of concentration camp survivors. *Applied Cognitive Psychology, 4,* 77-87.

Wagstaff, G. F. (1991). Compliance, belief, and semantics in hypnosis: A nonstate, sociocognitive perspective. Chapter in S. J. Lynn & J. W. Rhue (Eds.), *Theories of Hypnosis.* New York: Guilford, pp. 362-398.

Warren, A. R., & Swartwood, J. N. (1992). Developmental issues in flashbulb memory research: Children recall the Challenger event. Chapter in E. Winograd & U. Neisser (Eds.), *Affect and Accuracy in Recall: Studies of Flashbulb Memories.* New York: Cambridge University Press.

Watkins, J. G. (1949). *Hypnotherapy of War Neurosis.* New York: Ronald Press.

Watkins, J. G., & Watkins, H. H. (1979-1980). Ego states and hidden observers. *Journal of Altered States of Consciousness, 5,* 3-18.

Watkins, J. G., & Watkins, H. H. (1981). Ego state therapy. Chapter in R. Corsini (Ed.), *Handbook of Innovative Psychotherapies.* New York: Wiley, pp. 252-270.

Watkins, J. G. (1989). Hypnotic hypermnesia and forensic hypnosis: A cross-examination. *American Journal of Clinical Hypnosis, 32*(2), 71-83.

Watkins, J. G. (1992). *Hypnoanalytic Techniques.* New York: Irvington.

Watkins, J. G. (1993). Dealing with the problem of "false memory" in clinic and court. *Journal of Psychiatry & Law, 297-317.*

Weekes, J. R., Lynn, S. J., & Myers, B. (1993). Pseudomemory and hypnosis: The impact of stimulus factors. Unpublished manuscript, Ohio University. Cited in S. J. Lynn & M. R. Nash (1994), Truth in memory: Ramifications for psychotherapy and hypnotherapy, *American Journal of Clinical Hypnosis 36*(3), 194-208.

Weinberg, H. I., Wadsworth, J., & Baron, R. S. (1983). Demand and the impact of leading questions on eyewitness testimony. *Memory and Cognition, 11,* 101-104.

Weinberger, N. M., Gold, P.E., & Sternberg, D. B. (1984). Epinephrine enables Pavlovian fear conditioning under anesthesia. *Science, 223,* 605-607.

Weitzenhoffer, A. M. (1953). *Hypnotism: An Objective Study in Suggestibility.* New York: John Wiley.

Weitzenhoffer, A. M. (1989). *The Practice of Hypnotism, Vols. I & II.* New York: Wiley.

Weitzenhoffer, A. M., & Hilgard, E. R. (1962). *Stanford Hypnotic Susceptibility Scale, Form C.* Palo Alto: Consulting Psychologists Press.

Wells, G. L., & Leippe, M. R. (1981). How do people infer the accuracy of eyewitness identifications? Memory for peripheral detail can be misleading. *Journal of Applied Psychology, 66,* 682-687.

White, R. W., Fox, G. R., & Harris, W. W. (1940). Hypnotic hypermnesia for recently learned material. *Journal of Abnormal & Social Psychology, 35,* 88-103.

Whitehouse, W. G., Orne, E. C., Orne, M. T., & Dinges, D. F. (1991). Distinguishing the source of memories reported during prior waking and hypnotic recall attempts. *Applied Cognitive Psychology, 5,* 51-59.

Wickless, C., & Kirsch, I. (1989). The effects of verbal and experiential expectancy manipulations on hypnotic susceptibility. *Journal of Personality & Social Psychology, 57,* 762-768.

Wilkinson, C. B. (1983). Aftermath of a disaster: The collapse of the Hyatt Regency Hotel skywalks. *American Journal of Psychiatry, 140,* 1134-1139.

Williams, L. (1992). Adult memories of childhood abuse: Preliminary findings from a longitudinal study. *The Advisor, 5,* 19-20.

Wilson, L., Greene, E., & Loftus, E. F. (1986). Beliefs about forensic hypnosis. *International Journal of Clinical & Experimental Hypnosis, 34,* 110-121.

Wingfield, H. E. (1920). *An Introduction to the Study of Hypnotism.* London: Balliere Tindall.

Yuille, J. C. (1994). Personal correspondence to D. Corydon Hammond, August 9, 1994.

Yuille, J. C., & Cutshall, J. L. (1986). A case study of eyewitness memory of a crime. *Journal of Applied Psychology, 71*(2), 291-301.

Yuille, J. C., & Kim, C. K. (1987). A field study of the forensic use of hypnosis. *Canadian Journal of Behavioral Sciences Review, 19*(4), 418-429.

Yuille, J. C., & McEwan, N. H. (1985). Use of hypnosis as an aid to eyewitness memory. *Journal of Applied Psychology, 70*(2), 389-400.

Zaragoza, M. S., & Koshmidir, J. W. (1989). Misled subjects may know more than their performance implies. *Journal of Experimental Psychology: Learning, Memory, & Cognition, 15,* 246-255.

Zelig, M., & Beidelman, W. B. (1981). The investigative use of hypnosis. *International Journal of Clinical & Experimental Hypnosis, 29,* 401-412.